KIDS, SPORTS, AND CONCUSSION

Recent Titles in
The Praeger Series on Contemporary Health and Living

KIDS, SPORTS, AND CONCUSSION

A Guide for Coaches and Parents

WILLIAM PAUL MEEHAN, III, MD

The Praeger Series on Contemporary Health and Living
Julie K. Silver, Series Editor

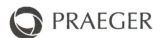 PRAEGER

AN IMPRINT OF ABC-CLIO, LLC
Santa Barbara, California • Denver, Colorado • Oxford, England

Library of Congress Cataloging-in-Publication Data

Meehan, William P.
  Kids, sports, and concussion : a guide for coaches and parents / William P. Meehan, III.
    p. cm. — (The Praeger series on contemporary health and living)
  Includes bibliographical references and index.
  ISBN 978–0–313–38730–2 (hardback) — ISBN 978–0–313–38731–9 (ebook)
1. Sports injuries in children. 2. Brain—Concussion. 3. Child athletes—Wounds and injuries. 4. Teenage athletes—Wounds and injuries. I. Title.
RC1218.C45M44   2011
617.4′81044083—dc22   2011004635

ISBN: 978–0–313–38730–2
EISBN: 978–0–313–38731–9

15 14 13 12 11   2 3 4 5

This book is also available on the World Wide Web as an eBook.
Visit www.abc-clio.com for details.

Praeger
An Imprint of ABC-CLIO, LLC

ABC-CLIO, LLC
130 Cremona Drive, P.O. Box 1911
Santa Barbara, California 93116-1911

This book is printed on acid-free paper ∞

Manufactured in the United States of America

For my wife, Marie

CONTENTS

SERIES FOREWORD

Over the past 100 years, there have been incredible medical breakthroughs that have prevented or cured illness in billions of people and helped many more improve their health while living with chronic conditions. A few of the most important twentieth-century discoveries include antibiotics, organ transplants, and vaccines. The twenty-first century has already heralded important new treatments including such things as a vaccine to prevent human papillomavirus from infecting and potentially leading to cervical cancer in women. Polio is on the verge of being eradicated worldwide, making it only the second infectious disease behind smallpox to ever be erased as a human health threat.

In this series, experts from many disciplines share with readers important and updated medical knowledge. All aspects of health are considered including subjects that are disease specific and preventive medical care. Disseminating this information will help individuals to improve their health as well as researchers to determine where there are gaps in our current knowledge and policy makers to assess the most pressing needs in healthcare.

Series Editor Julie K. Silver, MD
Assistant Professor
Harvard Medical School
Department of Physical Medicine and Rehabilitation

FOREWORD

I am very pleased to introduce Dr. Bill Meehan's parent's guide to sports-related concussions.

Such a book is long overdue. A true health crisis is emerging as we in the sports medicine field come to understand that far too many concussions are occurring on the sports field. What is even more disturbing is that this very dangerous injury is often not reported or is underreported. The short- and long-term implications of concussion injuries are not fully appreciated, and as a result, they are often managed in an inadequate fashion.

Dr. Meehan's book is the first book for parents on this subject. In this excellent resource you will find information that clarifies the extent of the concussion problem, signs you can use to recognize concussions in your own child, and proper guidelines for management, monitoring, and safe return to play for the young athlete.

Although sports medicine is a relatively young discipline, there is a growing awareness of how important it is that injuries sustained by athletes receive focused assessment and management. Injuries to young athletes are of particular concern. In addition to how we diagnose and treat these injuries, there is a particular emphasis now on injury *prevention*.

Nowhere is this more important than in sports injuries to the brain. Unlike other anatomical areas such as our bones, muscles, ligaments, and tendons, our brain tissue has relatively limited ability to heal and repair itself. If not recognized and treated early on, repeated injuries to the brain can result in lasting and permanent damage. And of course, above and beyond all other tissue in our body, the brain plays a fundamental role in our ability to function as human beings.

All this makes it imperative that we focus on early recognition and diagnosis of concussion injuries, especially in our children, who depend on us for their safety. Furthermore, everyone in the sports environment—parents, coaches, team officials, and athletes—must combine their efforts to find and implement the most effective means of *preventing* injuries to the young athlete's brain.

Dr. Meehan's book will explain to parents what your role is and will help you appreciate the wide-ranging impact of such an injury on your children's lives. This extends from their ability to interact with their peers, to completing homework assignments, all the way to their overall mood and behavior.

The great challenge for the next generation of sports medicine experts will be to develop systematic methods to prevent concussion in sports. This may include modified or new sports rules, coaches' and officials' education, and even new training techniques and protective equipment.

I believe every parent will find this new book a fascinating and comprehensive look at this important subject. I give it my highest recommendation and consider it a must-read in the growing lexicon of sports medicine books for a public interested in this field.

Lyle J. Micheli, MD
Director, Division of Sports Medicine, Children's Hospital Boston
O'Donnell Family Professor of Orthopedic Sports Medicine
Clinical Professor of Orthopedic Surgery, Harvard Medical School
Secretary General, International Federation of Sports Medicine
Past President, American College of Sports Medicine

ACKNOWLEDGMENTS

There are countless people I need to thank, not only for the production of this book, but for supporting me throughout my life and career. Without these people, I would not be in a position to do what I love, or to write a book about a topic that fascinates me. I have been blessed with people who supported and encouraged me in all of my pursuits.

William and Mary Meehan, my mother and father, remain a constant voice of encouragement and support. They always made the education of my sister and me their first priority. I quit my job in the mid-1990s, drained my savings account, and took out student loans in order to go back to college, take the medical prerequisite courses, and apply to medical school. But after the first day of chemistry class, I considered quitting. I hadn't taken a science class in five years. I could barely follow the lecture. I found the first homework assignment confusing, frustrating, and difficult. I questioned whether or not I could do it. I called home that evening, contemplating dropping out of the program. My mother convinced me to continue, however, just through the first test. As it turns out, I scored a solid A on the first test and never looked back.

In addition to their constant encouragement, my sister, Katie, her husband, Joe, my two nephews, Emmett and Patrick, and extended family members have all been supportive of my efforts throughout medical school, residency, two fellowships, and additional research training, despite my absence during many holidays, weddings, and family functions. This is especially noteworthy, as I come from an unusually close-knit extended family, on both my mother's and father's side. We spend every holiday together. Growing up, I saw my grandparents, aunts, uncles and cousins almost every weekend.

If it weren't for the counsel of my dear friend, Gina "Ma G" Story, I would have never even known that going to medical school was a possibility for someone who was not premed as an undergraduate. When I decided to pursue a career in medicine, I was working for the honorable Thomas M. Menino, mayor of the city of Boston. Mayor Menino and my immediate supervisor, current

Boston Chief of Policy and Planning, Michael J. Kineavy, were delighted and 100 percent supportive of my efforts.

When I interviewed for the fellowship in sports medicine at Children's Hospital Boston, I proposed to the Chief of the Division of Sports Medicine, Lyle J. Micheli, and the Fellowship Director, Pierre d'Hemecourt, that the division start a Sports Concussion Clinic. We started three weeks later, before I had even been accepted to the fellowship. Dr. d'Hemecourt served as cofounder of the clinic and has remained a constant supporter of the clinic and all its efforts. Dr. Micheli supplied all of the administrative and financial resources that are required to start such a program, allowing me to travel to other specialty clinics throughout the country to learn their approach to concussion management.

Since that time, the clinic has expanded dramatically. We currently see approximately 60 patients each week who suffer from concussive brain injury. The clinic includes several physicians, including Michael O'Brien, Andrea Stracciolini, and Pierre d'Hemecourt. We have a specialized nurse practitioner, Michelle Parker, who cares for all patients with traumatic brain injury throughout all of the various clinics in the hospital. We have a specialized nurse, Ariana Moccia, who works with each provider caring for athletes with concussions. Alex Taylor, a neuropsychologist with additional training in sport-related concussion, is our most recent addition. We are fortunate enough to have specialists in several medical and surgical specialties who work with us on special cases: Alyssa Lebel, Anna Minster, Mark Proctor, Ed Smith, Sharon Chirban, and Celiane Rey-Casserly. We have much needed administrative support from Kristen Hawkins, Soren Capawanna, Stacey Cobban, Maria Maginnis, and Maureen Piccolo.

We are assisted in clinical research by Chuck d'Hemecourt and Valerie Ugrinow, who coordinate all ongoing studies through the clinic. We have countless collaborators including Rebekah Mannix, Dawn Comstock, and Mickey Collins. Most of our projects are only possible because of the support, guidance, and teaching of clinical researchers Richard Bachur, Kenneth Mandl, Gary Fleisher, and the late Michael Shannon, who took an early interest in my career. I continue to rely on the guidance of Drs. Bachur and Mandl.

We are assisted in laboratory research by my teacher and mentor, pediatric intensivist Michael J. Whalen, and my colleagues in the lab, Rebekah Mannix, Jugta Khuman, Jimmy Zhang, Juyeon Park, Xiaoxia Zhu, and Jianhua Qiu.

When first learning how to best care for concussed athletes, I was fortunate enough to have guidance and support from more senior clinicians working in the field. Pierre d'Hemecourt served as a mentor and teacher from the start. I was allowed to observe neurosurgeon Robert Cantu, MD, and neuropsychologist, Mickey Collins, PhD, in their clinics. Both are world-famous leaders in the field of concussive brain injury in sports. They were kind enough to share their approaches to brain injury with me, and continue to support the efforts of our clinic.

With regards to this book, it resulted directly from discussions at Children's Hospital Boston with Lyle J. Micheli and Mark Jenkins, our division editor.

I proposed the idea to Dcb Carvalko, who saw the project through to completion, and provided much-needed direction for this first-time book author. It was edited with care and diligence by David Cocn.

The three athletes featured at the end of the book, Maggie Hickey, Sean Folan, and Nathan Kessel, were kind enough to share their personal stories with readers, giving insight into the effects of concussive brain injury on the lives of young scholar-athletes.

Most importantly, I must acknowledge the constant patience and support of my wife, Marie, who has allowed me to spend countless hours studying concussive brain injury, conducting clinical and scientific research, and preparing this book. She gave me the time I needed to dedicate to this book by keeping up our home and caring for our dog, Champ, in addition to holding her own full-time job. She found me a speech recognition software program to assist with the writing, as I am still a hunt-and-peck typist. She served as editor for the final draft that was submitted to the publishers, as she does for all of my medical manuscripts and other writings.

To each and every person noted above, I am truly grateful.

William Paul Meehan, III, MD

Introduction

We were in the heart of the rugby scrum. A 20-year-old lock playing for Boston College was struck in the head by the mighty kick of an opponent. As the ball was released, he staggered away toward the wrong end of the field before collapsing to the ground. He rose unsteadily, only to collapse again. Finally, he rose to his feet and began sprinting, in an attempt to rejoin the play. But he was running in the wrong direction, away from ball. He fell one last time, only to be helped off of the field by his teammates.

"What's the matter with him," hollered the coach.

"He's all right," came the reply. "He just got his bell rung."

And that was how it was.

We got "shaken up" or "had our bells rung." We simply "shook it off," "toughed it out," or "walked it off." The word *concussion* was rarely used. When it was used, it was mostly for athletes who were knocked unconscious for longer than a few seconds. Many times, we returned to the game in which we were injured. Often, we returned while still experiencing headaches, ringing in the ears, and other symptoms.

So why all the concern nowadays? What was it that changed the way sport-related concussion is diagnosed and managed? Why is the media constantly reporting stories about concussion in young athletes?

Five main medical findings change the way we think about sport-related concussion:

1. Concussion results in measurable brain dysfunction, which lasts for several days, weeks, or even months in some athletes.
2. This brain dysfunction often persists, even after the athlete reports being symptom-free.
3. Athletes who sustain one concussion are at increased risk of sustaining more-concussions in the future.

4. The effects of multiple concussions are cumulative.
5. There may be long-term effects, only revealed later in life, that result from sustaining multiple concussions earlier in an athlete's career.

These recent medical findings have led to a relatively rapid change in the way doctors and other clinicians think about sport-related concussions and concussive brain injury in general. This rapid change in thinking has generated a lot of attention, not only in the medical literature but also in the popular media. When many of us were growing up, a concussion was not thought to be a serious injury. Athletes often laughed and joked about it. Certainly few people believed that there were any long-term effects or brain dysfunction that could result from a concussion or even multiple concussions.

These days, we know that a concussion results in a true, measurable, loss of brain function, that can persist, even after athletes feel that they are completely recovered. Furthermore, we know that sustaining multiple concussions over the course of one's career can lead to more permanent brain dysfunction, depression, and other problems. This sudden change in thinking has left many athletes, parents, coaches, and others confused. This book will help clarify the medical and scientific data that has resulted in this change of thinking. In doing so, this book will answer the following questions:

• What is a concussion?
• How common is concussion?
• Can an athlete prevent a concussion?
• What is the best way to assess a concussion?
• What can be done to treat a concussion?
• When is it safe to return to playing after a concussion?
• What are the risks of suffering multiple concussions?

In addition, readers of this book will learn how they can respond to a concussed athlete, as well as what they should expect from medical personnel tending to a concussed athlete. For those readers interested in starting a comprehensive concussion management program in their area, this book contains some recommendations on how to proceed. Lastly, the book concludes with several athletes describing, in their own words, their experiences with concussions.

At the end of each chapter is a list of suggested readings for those readers who may wish to learn more about the topics covered within the chapter. Many of these readings are medical or scientific articles, often those referred to in the chapter. While these articles may use some medical and scientific jargon, I believe the overall principles can be appreciated, even without scientific or medical training.

1

DEFINITIONS AND TEAM MEMBERS: WHO WILL HELP CARE FOR THE ATHLETE WITH A SPORT-RELATED CONCUSSION?

Before we begin to look in depth at sport-related concussion in chapter 2, it will be helpful for the reader to be familiar with the names of the various medical personnel involved in assessing and managing sport-related concussions. Similarly, familiarity with certain terms that are used frequently in sports, sports medicine, and in the management of sport-related concussion will serve as an aid to understanding the chapters that follow.

PERSONNEL

Clinician

A general term for a medical professional who assesses and treats patients with an illness or injury. Doctors, nurses, psychologists, neuropsychologists, nurse practitioners, athletic trainers, physician assistants, and many others are all included under the term *clinician*.

Athletic Trainer (ATC)

A medically trained professional who specializes in the assessment and treatment sport related injuries. Often, a team will have its own athletic trainer or even several athletic trainers who oversee the healthcare of the team's athletes. When an athlete is injured, the athletic trainer is usually the first medical professional to respond. The athletic trainer will have the athlete explain how the injury occurred. The athletic trainer will examine the athlete and decide whether further management is needed. Often, the athletic trainer alone will treat the injury.

Athletic trainers have expertise in certain types of treatment, as well as in taping and bracing techniques, which can prevent injury or allow an athlete with a mild injury to continue to participate in sports. Athletic trainers are an essential part of the sports medicine team. Since their specialty is sport related injuries, athletic trainers, in general, will know as much, if not more, about sport-related concussion than other medical specialists who do not have an interest in sports medicine or concussive brain injury.

Sports Medicine Doctor

A doctor who has completed extra medical training focused on the illnesses and injuries of athletes, and how athletes are affected by illness and injury. Sports medicine doctors specialize in the assessment, management, and treatment of sport related injuries. There are two types of sports medicine doctors: sports medicine physicians and sports medicine surgeons.

Sports medicine surgeons are doctors who initially trained in orthopedic surgery and then went on to do specialty training in sport related surgery. They can perform many surgeries arthroscopically. That means, instead of cutting a joint open in order to reconstruct a ligament, repair an injured meniscus, or tend to other injured structures, they can make small incisions through which they insert a camera and other small tools needed for repairing or reconstructing injured structures. Such small incisions allow for quicker recovery times. Often, athletes who undergo arthroscopic surgery are able to return to sports sooner than those who undergo open surgeries. In addition to performing surgery, sports medicine surgeons are able to assess and treat many sport related injuries, mostly involving the bones, muscles, tendons and ligaments of athletes. Should an athlete sustain an injury which requires surgery, it is best performed by a sports medicine surgeon. Though not all surgeries can be performed arthroscopically, a surgeon trained in sports medicine will know which procedure is best for the athlete, allowing the athlete to safely return to play at his or her prior level of performance in the shortest possible amount of time.

Sports medicine physicians are doctors who initially trained in a medical field such as internal medicine, pediatrics, family practice, or emergency medicine. After their initial training, they went on to do more specialized training in the assessment and management of sport related injuries. While they will treat injuries related to bone, muscle, tendons, and ligaments, they will also treat many other illnesses suffered by athletes. As sport-related concussion is a common injury in athletes, these physicians will be educated and knowledgeable about the assessment and management of sport-related concussions.

Team Physician

A doctor who is dedicated to work with a specific athletic team. For professional, college, and many other teams with significant resources, this doctor will almost always be one who is trained in sports medicine. However, for those teams without such resources, this may be a physician or an orthopedic surgeon who has an interest in sports and takes care of the athletes without having any specific training in sports medicine. Frequently, the team physician manages not only the athletic injuries of the team but also other common ailments and illnesses that arise throughout the season, such as influenza outbreaks and chronic conditions, such as asthma, that might affect a team's athletes.

Neuropsychologist

A scientist and clinician who specializes in the assessment of brain function. Neuropsychologists have earned either a doctor of psychology degree (PsyD) or a doctor of philosophy degree (PhD). When a neuropsychologist sees a patient, he or she will ask the patient to perform certain tasks to help the neuropsychologist measure elements of brain function. In the setting of sport-related concussion, neuropsychologists are used for several purposes. Sometimes, they will administer neuropsychological tests prior to the start of the sports season in order to obtain what is known as a baseline measurement of brain function. These are measurements of brain function in the healthy athlete. They can be used later if necessary to assess changes in brain function should a concussive injury occur. In addition, neuropsychologists are called upon to measure brain function after injury, to help determine whether an athlete has sustained a sport-related concussion and to provide strategies to help athletes during recovery from such injuries. For those athletes who are unfortunate enough to have a slow recovery from their sport-related concussions, the neuropsychologist will often use measurements of brain function to help determine the athlete's abilities. A neuropsychologist may assist with devising an academic plan to help the athlete learn while recovering brain function resulting from the injury.

Nurse Practitioner (NP)

A nurse who has gone on to do extra medical training. Nurse practitioners are able to evaluate patients, order tests, make diagnoses, and prescribe treatments for those diagnoses, including medications. They act, in many ways, like physicians. But they have not undergone the same training as a doctor and do not have an MD degree.

Physician Assistant (PA or PA-C for Physician Assistant, Certified)

Like a nurse practitioner, a physician assistant has completed medical training that allows him or her to evaluate patients, order tests, make diagnoses, and prescribe treatments for those diagnoses, including medications. A physician assistant acts in many ways like a physician but has not undergone the same training as a doctor and does not have an MD degree.

Primary Care Physician

The doctors that most readers will be familiar with. These physicians have trained in internal medicine, pediatrics, or family practice. Unlike sports medicine physicians, these doctors have not completed extra medical training in the assessment and management of sport related injuries. However, many will take an active interest in managing athletes. Some of these physicians will be up to date on the current medical literature regarding sport-related concussion. Some will have all the available resources to properly treat young athletes. It is these physicians who provide care to most athletes who sustain sport-related concussions. If sport-related concussion is not an injury that a certain primary care physician is confident managing, or if a particular athlete or injury is medically complicated, the primary care physician may consult with other doctors who have more specialized training in the assessment and management of sport-related concussions or concussive brain injuries in general.

Neurosurgeon

A surgeon who specializes in performing operations on the skull, brain, spine, and spinal cord. Although concussion is not an injury that requires surgery, many neurosurgeons will be familiar with the assessment and management of concussions. Many will manage athletes with concussion. Those who do not will likely be familiar with other clinicians in their local area who manage sport-related concussions.

Neurologist

A doctor who specializes in the diseases and illnesses that affect the nerves of the body and brain. Although concussive brain injury is not typically a part of neurology training, some neurologists will have taken an active interest in this area and can assess and manage a sport-related concussion. Often, these highly skilled physicians will be called upon to assist in the management of post-concussive headaches, or headaches that occur after a concussion. At Children's Hospital Boston, we are fortunate to have several neurologists with an interest in concussive brain injury.

Psychologist/Sports Psychologist

A clinician who specializes in treating emotional disturbances and behavioral problems. The psychologist or sports psychologist offers therapy via counseling and is often able to provide strategies to help athletes manage emotional and behavioral problems. A sports psychologist is a psychologist who has taken specialized training and has an active interest in those psychological problems that affect athletes and athletic performance. In the realm of sport-related concussion, sports psychologists help athletes cope with their injuries and the limitations on their life that result from concussive brain injury.

Psychiatrist

A physician who specializes in the assessment and management of mental illness. In the realm of sport-related concussions, a psychiatrist may be consulted to help manage the depression experienced by some athletes who suffer a prolonged recovery after sustaining a sport-related concussion. These cases are rare. For most athletes recovering from a sport-related concussion, psychiatric medications will not be indicated.

School Nurse

Often one of the first clinicians to assess an athlete who has sustained a sport-related concussion. Some schools are not fortunate enough to have an athletic trainer. Other times, the athletic trainer may be unavailable, as when he or she is on the road with a team that has an away game. Therefore, athletes injured during a home game may be taken to the school nurse. As sport-related concussions draw more and more attention both in the medical literature and in the popular media, school nurses are being called upon more frequently to help coordinate the assessment and management of sport-related concussions.

TERMS

Cognitive Function

Cognitive is a medical term used to describe certain functions of the brain. Cognitive function refers to those functions of the brain that involve thinking, concentrating, learning, and reasoning. Throughout much of the medical literature, the terms *cognitive, neurocognitive,* and *neuropsychological* are often used interchangeably. While there are, in fact, subtle differences in their meaning, the terms may be considered relative for the sake of this text. Often, *brain function* will be used as a generic term to describe overall cognitive function. Tasks that require cognitive effort include: reading, studying, videogame playing, working online, text messaging, playing games such as chess or Scrabble, and other similar activities.

Signs

Medical professionals often refer to the *signs* and *symptoms* of an illness or injury. The *signs* of an illness or injury are those characteristics that can be observed by people other than the patient. For example, a rash would be a *sign* of illness. Swelling would be a *sign* of injury.

Symptoms

The characteristics of an injury or illness that are experienced by patients themselves. Nausea, for example, would be a *symptom* of an illness. Pain would be a *symptom* of an injury.

Amnesia

A medical term referring to a loss of memory, often caused by a traumatic injury to the brain.

Cervical Spine

Term used collectively for the seven smaller bones of the spine that are located within the neck. As opposed to being one long bone, the spine, or backbone, consists of multiple small bones stacked on top of one another. The cervical spine, houses and protects the spinal cord, a set of nerves descending from the brain that control much of our bodily movements and sensations. Damage to the cervical spine can also result in damage to the spinal cord. This can lead to devastating consequences, including death and paralysis.

Noncontact Sports

Sports in which contact with another player is neither an intentional nor an expected part of the game. Some common noncontact sports include tennis, cross-country running, track and field, and swimming.

Contact Sports

Sports in which contact with another player is an expected part of the game. However, intentional blows to the body are not routinely delivered. Common contact sports are soccer, basketball, and baseball. The meaning of this term is often unclear. Some will refer to both basketball and ice hockey as contact sports. However, it will be apparent to most readers that the frequency of contact, the force of contact, and the intensity of contact that occurs during basketball is quite different than that which occurs during ice hockey. Therefore, in this book, we divide sports into three main categories: contact, noncontact, and collision. (A fourth type of sport, combat, is categorized as a subset of collision).

Collision Sports

Sports in which intentional body-to-body blows are part of the game. Common collision sports include American football, ice hockey, rugby, and lacrosse.

Combat Sports

A subset of collision sports. Most combat sports are one-on-one contests in which two combatants are engaged in a fight, albeit with a specific set of rules and regulations that are followed and monitored by a referee. Common combat sports are boxing, wrestling, karate, mixed martial arts and other similar activities.

Trauma

A wound or injury caused by a blow, collision, or force. Common examples of traumatic injuries are fractures, gunshot wounds, lacerations, bruises, and concussions.

Concussive Brain Injury

Another term for concussion. Concussive brain injury refers to an injury to the brain that, as we shall see, results from a rapid spinning or rotational acceleration of the brain.

Traumatic Brain Injury

An injury to the brain that results from trauma, as defined above. There are other ways that the brain can be injured. For example, if one has an arterial blood clot and blood cannot flow to the brain, the brain will sustain an injury from this lack of blood flow. Such an injury is more commonly referred to as a "stroke." This type of injury, however, is not due to trauma. When we discuss concussion, we are referring to a specific type of traumatic brain injury.

Mild Traumatic Brain Injury (mTBI)

A term often used interchangeably with *concussion*. However, as many patients will attest, concussions are often far from mild. The term mild does not describe how significant the patient's symptoms can be or how long it can take the patient to recover.

Furthermore, while the terms *concussion* and *concussive brain injury* describe how the injury occurred (that it resulted, as defined above, from a rapid spinning or rotational acceleration). The term *mild traumatic brain injury* does not specify the way in which the injury occurred. In fact, the classification *mild traumatic brain injury* is solely determined by how the patient appears to the doctor at the time of presentation. It is based on an evaluation of head trauma known as the Glasgow Coma Scale, or GCS. The Glasgow Coma Scale is used by emergency medicine providers to communicate the level of consciousness of a patient who has sustained a trauma. The patient is given a number of points based on his or her response to various stimuli. Table 1.1 shows a version of the Glasgow Coma Scale, using common terminology.

Table 1.1
A Modified Version of the Glasgow Coma Scale.

	Glasgow Coma Scale	
Motor response	The patient obeys commands	6
	The patient responds to a painful stimulus by moving toward the site of the stimulus	5
	The patient moves away from the a painful stimulus	4
	The patient flexes his or her joints in response to a painful stimulus	3
	The patients extends his or her joints in response to a painful stimulus	2
	The patient has no response to a painful stimulus	1
Verbal response	The patient is able to respond appropriately to questions regarding who he or she is and where he or she is	5
	The patient responds to questions, but is confused	4
	The patient responds to questioning using inappropriate words. There is no conversation	3
	The patient makes incomprehensible sounds, but no actual words	2
	No response to questioning	1
Eye opening	The patient spontaneously opens his or her eyes	4
	The patient opens his or her eyes to speech	3
	The patients opens his or her eyes to painful stimulus	2
	The patients does not open his or her eyes, despite painful stimulus	1
Total possible score		15

Patients with suspected concussive injury are categorized as having mild traumatic brain injury if, when they arrive for medical care, they have a total score of 14–15 on the Glasgow Coma Scale. An uninjured person would typically have a score of 15.

While highly useful in the sphere of emergency response to trauma, the Glasgow Coma Scale should not be used to assess the significance of a concussion. It does not predict how long it will take an athlete to recover from a concussion. Many patients who are diagnosed with mild traumatic brain injury have diminished brain function, headaches, and other symptoms that last weeks or even months. Alternatively, some patients diagnosed with "moderate" traumatic brain injury will recover completely within days to weeks. Therefore, the term *mild traumatic brain injury* should not be used interchangeably with *concussion*. Readers should understand that athletes will recover from most concussions rapidly, within hours or days. Other concussions, however, will result in symptoms that last months. At present, it is not possible to accurately predict which injuries will resolve rapidly and which will result in more prolonged recovery.

SUGGESTED READINGS

Bailes, J., *Sports-Related Concussion.* 1999, St. Louis, MO: Quality Medical Publishing.

Echemendia, R. J., *Sports Neuropsychology: Assessment and Management of Traumatic Brain Injury.* 2006, New York: The Guilford Press.

Lee, L. K., Consequences of the Sequelae of Pediatric Mild Traumatic Brain Injury. *Pediatr Emerg Care,* 2007. 23(8): 580–86.

Lovell, M. R., R. E. Echemendia, J. T. Barth, and M. W. Collins, *Traumatic Brain Injury in Sports: An International Neuropsychological Perspective.* 2004, Lisse, The Netherlands: Swets and Zeitlinger.

McCrea, M., *Mild Traumatic Brain Injury and Postconcussion Syndrome: The New Evidence Base for Diagnosis and Treatment.* 2008, New York: Oxford University Press.

Nowinski, C., *Head Games: Football's Concussion Crisis.* 2007, East Bridgewater, MA: The Drummond Publishing Group.

2

WHAT IS A CONCUSSION?

On October 30, 1974, the world heavyweight champion, George Foreman, fought Muhammad Ali in a bout that will forever be remembered as the "rumble in the jungle." Many readers my age or older will remember watching this fight on television or seeing the countless replays of it over the last 36 years. The fight was memorable for many reasons. It was only the second time in heavyweight history that a former champion reclaimed the title. It introduced Don King to the world as a professional boxing promoter. The fight took place in Zaire, in central Africa, a country now known as the Democratic Republic of Congo. It ended with controversy as some argue that Foreman was counted out despite being on his feet by the count of nine. But perhaps the "rumble in the jungle" is most remembered for the strategy Ali used during the fight, which has come to be known as "rope a dope."

Early in the fight, Ali began lying against the ropes, allowing George Foreman to deliver multiple blows. He mounted few attacks against the reigning champion. He dodged many of Foreman's thrusts. He blocked many aside. He allowed several of the less powerful blows to land on relatively harmless areas of the body. He tangled Foreman up, and wrestled with him. He taunted Foreman, challenging him to throw harder, more vicious blows. Foreman, who was recognized as the more powerful fighter, seemed only too happy to oblige. As the fight went on, however, the amount of energy Foreman spent in trying to land these powerful blows, and trying to disentangle himself from Ali, took its toll. He was visibly tired at the start of the eighth round.

In fact, the beginning if not most of the eighth round seemed little different from the prior rounds. Ali allowed Foreman to punch away, only occasionally offering a quick straight jab to Foreman's face. But as the round neared its end, with only 18 seconds remaining, Ali unleashed a flurry of blows. In the final combination, Ali stood Foreman nearly upright with a left hook to the face. Foreman's left hand dropped to his side, exposing his chin to a punishing right cross that Ali landed squarely on Foreman's jaw. With only 12 seconds remaining in the round, Foreman, staggered, fell, and was counted out, ending the fight.

George Foreman had been concussed.

But why? What is it that happened to George Foreman's brain at the time of that right cross that rendered him stunned, off balance, incapable of continuing the fight? What was it about that right cross that resulted in Foreman's brain malfunctioning? If the brain is located in the top of the head, above the eyes, why would a punch to the jaw injure the brain at all? This chapter will provide answers to these questions.

A concussion is a type of traumatic brain injury. When athletes sustain concussions, their brains stop functioning properly as a result of trauma. Perhaps the simplest way to think of a sport-related concussion is as a temporary dysfunction of the brain caused by trauma.

Despite popular belief, a concussion is not a bruise on the brain. There is no detectable bruising, bleeding, or swelling of the brain. It is not cut, scratched, or abraded. However, the brain cannot function properly when it is concussed. Memory, concentration, reaction time, the ability to learn new information, and the ability to solve problems are all temporarily damaged when an athlete sustains a concussion.

Since one of the main functions of the brain is to maintain consciousness, any athlete who loses consciousness after head trauma has sustained a concussion. However, most concussions in sports do not involve a loss of consciousness. In fact, less than 10 percent of all sport-related concussions involve a loss of consciousness.

A blow dealt to the shoulder will bruise the shoulder. Most people are familiar with this type of injury. Therefore, many people believe that a concussion is a bruise on the brain sustained by a blow to the head. Medical science, however, has shown that this is not true. Remember, the brain is protected by the thick, hard bone of the skull. In order to bruise the brain, the skull would have to break or bend inward and strike the brain. While this can happen, the forces involved in sports are often too low to cause this type of skull deformity. Furthermore, in the sports that result in the most concussions, the brain is often protected by a hard helmet in addition to the skull. In fact, many concussions are caused by a blow to the face mask, or other part of the body, as opposed to the head. Readers who are familiar with boxing or mixed martial arts will be well aware of this. Concussions are fairly common in these sports. For a physician who studies concussive brain injury, a lot can be learned from observing these combat sports.

Just the other evening I was having trouble sleeping. I got out of bed, went into the living room, and began watching some television. I came across a show featuring the ultimate fighting championship's (UFCs) greatest knockouts. I started watching volume 3. I was on volume 6 by the time I returned to bed. There were approximately five or six knockouts per episode. So I was able to observe a good number of concussions in a relatively short period of time.

I noticed that most of these knockouts resulted from a blow to the chin. Remember that the brain is in the top of the skull, mostly above the eyes. A blow to the chin results in no impact on the brain whatsoever. However, it does result in a significant movement or "spinning" of the brain at the time of impact. As we shall soon see, it is this rapid movement of the brain that results in a concussion.

So what is it that causes a concussion?

A concussion is caused by an acceleration of the brain. After the head, face, or other part of the body is struck, the brain is sent spinning in the opposite direction. For example, if a basketball player is struck on the left side of the face by the elbow of an opponent, his or her head will accelerate to the right. This rapid movement, or acceleration, of the brain causes it to malfunction. In particular, rotational acceleration or spinning of the brain results in injury.

There are two ways to accelerate something. You can push it in a straight line, such that it accelerates in a straight line, away from your pushing hand. This type of acceleration is known as linear acceleration. Imagine a car at a stoplight along a straight road. When the light turns green, the driver steps on the gas. The car goes from a complete stop, and accelerates, in a straight line, until the driver reaches a cruising speed at 25–30 miles per hour. This is a form of linear acceleration.

Alternatively, you can accelerate something by spinning it. "Spinning" is a more common term for rotational acceleration. When a child takes a toy top or dreidel, places it on a table, and spins it, the child is, in scientific terms, applying a rotational acceleration to the top. It is this rotational type of acceleration that results in concussion. This has been demonstrated in scientific experiments carried out over the last century.

In some sense, it has been known for over 100 years that in order to sustain a concussion, the head has to be free to move. As often happens, this was first realized in the world outside of medicine. This knowledge was commonly used in slaughterhouses. In order to prepare various meats for market the animals must first be killed. This takes place in slaughterhouses. It was thought inhumane to simply walk up to the animal and kill it. Therefore, men who worked in slaughter houses used to try and stun the animal or knock it unconscious prior to killing it and butchering it in preparation for the market. One common method used to stun the animal was to deliver a concussion by striking it on the head with a bolt. Certainly, if the animal's head was held in place, preventing it from moving, it would be quite easy to strike it with the bolt. By holding the head still, the butcher could maintain the head in precisely the location where the bolt would be striking from above. However, the men working in the slaughter houses knew that if the animal's head was held in place, and not free to move, the animal would not be stunned. It would not be concussed. It would not lose consciousness. However, if the animal was held in place by the shoulders and torso, so that the head was free to move after it was struck by the bolt, the animal would often be concussed. Once the animal was stunned from its concussion, the business of the day could proceed.

In the 1940s, this realization came to the medical community. Two research-ers named Denny-Brown and Russell, were studying concussion in animals. In order to concuss the animals, they would strike them in the head with a weight attached to a pendulum. The weight would be dropped from various heights, swing downward, and strike the animal in the head. From their experiments we have learned that if the head is held in place, and not allowed to move after it is struck, there are cuts or lacerations of the scalp, sometimes broken skull bones, and sometimes bleeding in the brain. The brain, however, seems to func-tion properly. The animal is upset and angry, but does not appear stunned, dazed, disoriented, and is seldom not knocked unconscious. If, however, the head is free to move after it has been struck, the brain stops functioning prop-erly. The animals often lose consciousness or "get knocked out." When they are not knocked unconscious, they are clearly off balance and dazed. This led physicians and scientists to believe that it was not the blow itself that causes a concussion but rather the rapid movement of the brain after the blow.

Over time, other medical and scientific research confirmed these findings. In order to sustain a concussion, the head must be free to move. The head must accelerate after impact in order for a concussion to occur. This led doctors and scientists to conclude that it is the acceleration of the brain which leads to a concussion as opposed to the impact itself. But whether it was linear acceleration or rotational acceleration that led to the injury remained unknown.

Around that same time, some other observations were made. The brain con-sists mostly of water. Perhaps as a result, many of the physical properties of the brain are similar to those of water. For a moment, think about what would hap-pen to a bowl of water with feathers floating on top if you were to slide it along a slippery surface, such as a piece of ice. By sliding it, you would be, in scientific terms, applying a linear acceleration to it. Once the bowl stopped sliding, the feathers would bob up and down on top of the waves. But the relative positions of the feathers to one another would remain the same. Each feather would remain in more or less in the same place within the bowl, bobbing up and down on top of the waves. If, however, you were to spin the bowl instead of sliding it in a straight line, feathers would be thrown around the bowl ending up in vari-ous locations. By spinning it, you would be, in scientific terms, applying a rota-tional acceleration to it.

A similar thought experiment was carried out by a physicist named Holburn in the 1940s. In order to follow up on this thought experiment, Holburn made a gelatin model of the brain, a fake brain made of a substance similar to Jell–O. He put this gelatin brain inside a wax model of a skull. He then spun the skull and brain, or, in scientific terms, he applied a rotational acceleration to the skull and brain. He then cracked open the wax skull and removed the fake brain. He saw extensive damage to it. He described the location of the damage sustained by his gelatin brain and published his findings in a medical journal known as the *Lancet.* This led him as well as other scientists and physicians to believe that "spinning" a brain, caused more damage than simply accelerating it in a straight line. However, the debate over whether rotational acceleration of the brain was more harmful than linear acceleration continued for some time.

More than thirty years after Holburn's experiment, the debate was taken up again. In order to better determine the effects of linear and rotational acceleration on the brain, two scientists, named Ommaya and Gennarelli, took the experiments one step further. They produced concussion without ever striking the brain. They separated 24 monkeys into two groups. Each monkey had a helmet snugly affixed to its head. For 12 of the monkeys, they used a mechanical device, to move the helmet rapidly forward, in a straight line, one inch. All of the monkeys who underwent this linear acceleration of one inch appeared fine afterward. They did not appear confused, off balance, or dazed. They did not lose consciousness.

The remaining 12 monkeys were placed in helmets as well. But this time, the helmets were spun or rotated over an arc of one inch, using the exact same amount of force. This rapid rotational acceleration resulted in all 12 monkeys being immediately knocked unconscious. Note, there was no blow to the brain; the animals were not struck in any way. Thus, this experiment confirmed that it was not simply the rapid movement or acceleration of the brain that produced the concussion but rather the spinning or "rotational acceleration" which resulted in concussive brain injury.

More recently, video analysis of concussions and studies performed on players from the National Football League revealed that most concussive injuries are caused when a player is struck on the side of the helmet or face mask. In fact, the face mask often acts as fulcrum, with face mask blows causing a more rapid acceleration of the brain than blows to the shell of the helmet. Such a blow results in a rotational acceleration of the brain, or spinning of the brain, in the opposite direction from the blow.

In many ways, a blow to the facemask and a blow to the chin result in a similar action on the brain. Let us consider for a moment a boxer striking one of his opponents. If a powerful blow is landed in the middle of the head, say just above the left ear, it may cause a lateral bending of the neck. The neck may be stretched, such that the boxer's head bends down toward the right, with the right ear moving down toward the right shoulder. If, however, the boxer throwing the punch manages to land his blow on the chin, side of the face, or side of his opponent's forehead, the head of the boxer struck will spin very rapidly toward the right. Thus, the athlete struck more toward the front of the head is more likely to sustain a concussion than the athlete struck in the middle of the head. Those of you seeking confirmation for this need merely watch ultimate fighting championships greatest knockouts, YouTube videos of fights that result in knockouts, or ESPN's classic bouts in which one of the boxers is knocked out.

The facemask extends even farther from the center of the head toward the front of the athlete. As with a boxer, if a football player is struck in the center of his helmet, say just above the left ear hole, again the head will bend down toward the opposite shoulder. Its acceleration will be restrained somewhat by the neck musculature, which will resist bending in that direction. If, however, the football player is struck on the front of his face mask, the head will spin very rapidly in the opposite direction. Therefore, a blow dealt to the front of the helmet or facemask is more likely to result in a concussion than a blow dealt to the center of the helmet.

It should be pointed out that, while rotational acceleration or spinning of the brain leads to a concussion, the spinning may occur in multiple different directions. For example, imagine a boxer who is struck by an uppercut. If the uppercut lands directly on the under surface of his chin, his head will spin upward, such that his face accelerates from its starting position, facing his opponent, upward, so that ultimately he is facing the ceiling. Thus, his head accelerates or spins in an upward direction. If, however, that same boxer is struck by a right cross that lands on his left cheek, his head would spin over his right shoulder. As opposed to spinning upward, his head would be spinning toward the right. In either case, he could sustain a concussion. So long as the brain is spinning—accelerating in a rotational fashion—a concussion can occur.

In life, most blows to the head result in rotational accelerations in several directions. It is rare for an uppercut to land directly in the center of the chin, accelerating the brain perfectly upward. More often the blow is landed on the side of the chin, which accelerates the brain upward but also off to the side. Similarly, in most real-life situations, there is both a linear and a rotational acceleration present. However, as noted, it is the rotational component of the acceleration that causes the concussion.

So, now we know that concussion is caused by a rotational acceleration, or "spinning," of the brain. But what happens to the brain, when it is spun, that prevents it from working properly?

To understand that, we must understand a little bit about how the brain works. But first, it will help us to consider a common, everyday, phenomenon that is analogous to the workings of the brain cells. Many readers will be familiar with what happens to a rope when one end is raised, and then rapidly lowered. An upside down U shape appears in the rope, and travels down its length, until it reaches the end. In this way, an "impulse" can be transmitted from one end of a rope, to the other end (Figure 2.1).

In some sense, the cells of the brain work similarly.

The brain consists of a collection of special cells, called nerve cells or "neurons." These nerve cells control all of our movements, thoughts, and bodily functions such as breathing. Each nerve cell consists of a cell body and an axon. The axon is a long, narrow part of the nerve cell used to transmit messages to other parts of the brain and other parts of the body. Nerve cells work,

Figure 2.1
Impulse Movement Along the Length of a Rope.

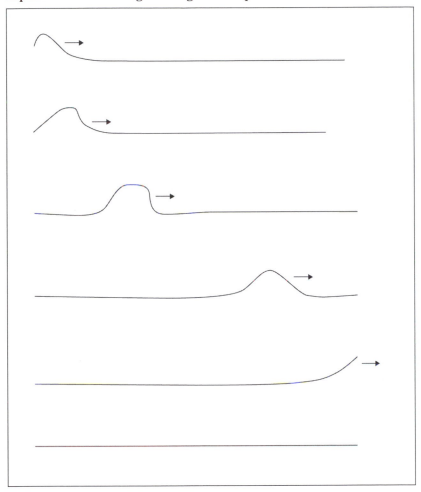

in part, by the movement of small molecules, called electrolytes. Most athletes will be familiar with the electrolytes sodium and potassium, which are commonly lost through sweat and replaced by sports drinks such as Gatorade. Movement of these electrolytes along the nerve cells is essential for normal brain function.

Usually sodium and potassium are on opposite sides of the outer lining of the cell called the cell membrane (Figure 2.2). Specifically, sodium is on the outside; potassium is on the inside. In a normal functioning neuron, the cell can conduct messages down its axon by movement of these electrons across

Figure 2.2
A Neuron Conducting a Message.

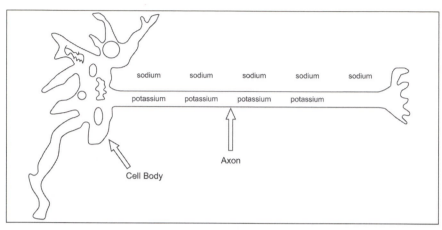

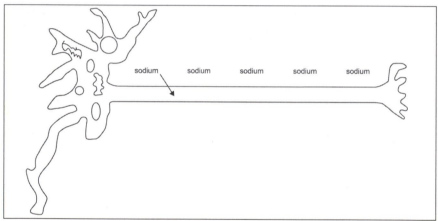

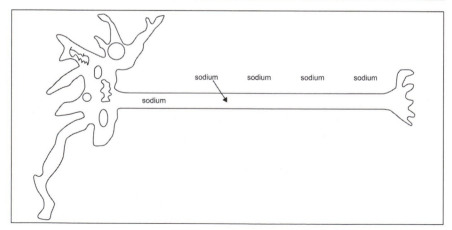

Figure 2.2 Continued

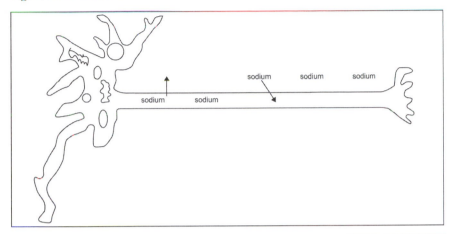

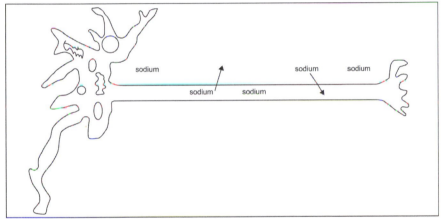

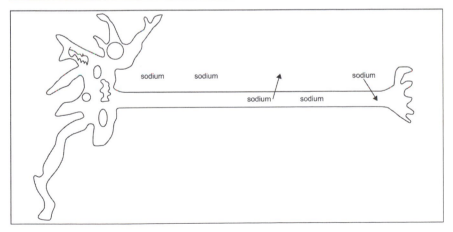

Figure 2.2 Continued

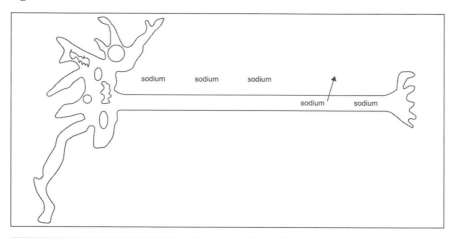

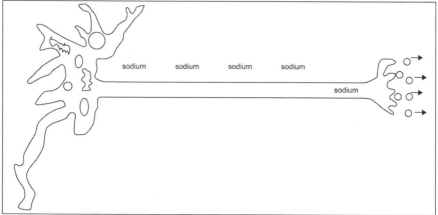

its membrane. When stimulated, a nerve cell will allow sodium to move into the cell from the outside (Figure 2.2). When this occurs at the start of the axon, it stimulates the adjacent area to do the same: allow sodium in. Very rapidly, however the sodium is pumped back to the outside of the cell. As sodium is moving into the cell at one part of the axon, it is being returned to the outside of the cell in the previous part of the axon. This occurs all the way down the length of the axon. Thus, this "impulse" is transmitted rapidly down the length of the axon, much like the impulse started on the rope discussed above is transported all the way down the length of the rope. When the person holding the rope raises and lowers it rapidly, he or she creates an impulse that transmits down the length of the rope. As one portion of the rope rises from its resting position, the other part of the rope returns to where it was previously.

Although, I am sure it seems complicated when reading about it in a paragraph, a picture is often worth a thousand words. Figures 2.1 and 2.2 should go a long way in helping to understand this concept.

When this exchange of ions across the membrane, or "impulse," reaches the end of the neuron, a chemical is secreted, sending a message to the next neuron.

That is how the brain normally functions. But, when an athlete sustains a concussion, the locations of sodium and potassium are disrupted. Large amounts of sodium move into the cell, while potassium moves out of the cell. Because such large amounts move across the membrane, it takes a long time to restore them to the proper positions. The nerve cell cannot operate normally until the sodium and potassium ions are put back in their normal place. During this time, the brain is concussed. It cannot function properly. In order to restore sodium and potassium to their normal positions along the cell membrane, the brain needs energy. Normally, energy is delivered to the brain through the bloodstream. Ironically, some experiments show that there is decreased blood flow to the brain after it has sustained a concussion. Thus, the brain receives less energy, at a time when it needs more energy. It is believed that this mismatch, between the need for more energy and the delivery of less energy, results in some of a patient's post-concussion symptoms.

Knowing a little bit about how the brain works is helpful. But how can you tell if an athlete has sustained a concussion?

Concussion can be detected by various *signs* and *symptoms*. Symptoms are the feelings or problems experienced by an athlete who has sustained a concussion. Common symptoms of concussion are headaches, nausea, difficulty balancing, difficulty concentrating, and amnesia (the inability to remember things that occurred around the time of injury). Some of the most common symptoms of concussion are listed in Table 2.1.

In addition to the symptoms experienced by the athlete, **signs** of concussion may be noticed by coaches, parents, and teammates. **Signs** are observations made by others, about an athlete who has sustained a concussion. Common signs seen in athletes who have sustained a concussion are poor balance or coordination, running the wrong play, vomiting, appearing glassy-eyed, seeming confused, or asking the same question over and over again despite being given the answer previously. Some of the common signs of concussion are listed in Table 2.2.

In order to help athletic trainers, doctors, and other medical personnel assess these signs and symptoms, standard lists have been developed. An athlete who has sustained an injury can rank these symptoms on what is known as a "symptom scale," or "symptom inventory." Symptom scales are often used to monitor an athlete's recovery. The Sports Concussion Assessment Tool version 2 (SCAT 2) contains a common symptom scale used by the International Olympic Committee, the Fédération Internationale de Football Association (FIFA), International Rugby Board, and International Ice Hockey Federation. The SCAT 2 is included in the appendix, at the end of this book.

Table 2.1
Common Symptoms of a Sport-Related Concussion.

Symptoms of Concussion

- Headache
- Dizziness
- Difficulty concentrating
- Nausea or vomiting
- Difficulty balancing
- Vision changes
- Sensitivity to light
- Sensitivity to noise
- Feeling "out of it"
- Ringing in the ears
- Drowsiness
- Sadness

People often wonder whether there are tests that can be performed to determine for sure whether or not an athlete has a concussion. While there are no perfect tests for concussion, there are some that can help determine whether or not an athlete has sustained a concussion. Some of these tests are used to assess whether or not there is another reason that might explain the athlete's symptoms. These tests should be normal if the athlete's symptoms are due to

Table 2.2
Common Signs of a Sport-Related Concussion.

Symptoms of Concussion

- Loss of consciousness
- Amnesia, or forgetfulness
- Walking off-balance
- Acting disoriented
- Appearing dazed
- Acting confused
- Forgetting game rules or play assignments
- Inability to recall score or opponent
- Inappropriate emotionality
- Poor physical coordination
- Slow verbal responses
- Personality changes

a concussion. Other tests are used to determine the degree to which an athlete's brain has been concussed. These tests will often be abnormal after an athlete sustains a concussion.

Many readers will be familiar with pictures of the brain or medical images such as computed tomogram (CT) scans or magnetic resonance images (MRIs). CT scans and MRIs are similar to X-rays. They are types of pictures used by doctors to help determine whether or not a body part, such as the brain, has sustained a structural injury. These pictures can often tell whether or not a body part has been bruised, broken, lacerated, swollen, or sustained other traumatic injury. Unlike an X-ray, these pictures allow doctors to see soft tissues, such as the brain, in addition to bone.

As there is no bruising, bleeding, or swelling of the brain when an athlete sustains a concussion, CT scans and MRIs of the brain will be normal. A doctor cannot "see" a concussion by looking at these images. Often, these types of images will be ordered by the doctor in order to make sure there is not another injury, in addition to the concussion, which explains some of the athlete's symptoms. They are very useful in making sure the athlete does not have bleeding in the brain, swelling of the brain, or a skull fracture. Many times, however, these types of images will not be necessary.

Similarly, there is no blood test or other type of medical test that can definitively diagnose a concussion. Several possible blood tests have been studied by medical researchers. However, as of the time of this writing, none has proved effective in definitively diagnosing a concussive brain injury. Currently, at Children's Hospital Boston, there is medical research being conducted in order to identify tests from the blood, tests from the urine, tests of the cerebral spinal fluid, and other types of pictures or images which may help doctors definitively diagnose concussive brain injury. Until such tests have been discovered, doctors must rely, in part, on athletes reporting their symptoms to us. As many athletes do not understand concussion, or even recognize a concussion when it occurs, they often do not report their symptoms. Furthermore, many who do recognize that their symptoms are due to a concussion are so anxious to get back to play that they pretend to feel better in order to get cleared for participation. Thus, it can often be difficult to determine whether or not an athlete has sustained a concussion. It can be even more challenging to determine when exactly an athlete has recovered from a concussion.

Fortunately, there are some tests which can be helpful in determining whether or not athlete has sustained a concussion as well as when an athlete has recovered from a concussion. There are standard ways of measuring athletes balance. The neurological physical examination may reveal certain findings which are inconsistent with concussion and may cause doctors to look for other potential causes of an athlete's signs or symptoms. Brain function can be measured. Neuropsychological or neurocognitive tests measure brain function. Each of these tests can be used to assist clinicians in diagnosing a concussion. They will be discussed in detail in later chapters.

It is understandably frustrating for doctors, parents, coaches, and athletes that no medical test can definitively diagnose a concussion. Many of the symptoms of concussion can also be caused by other medical conditions. For example, headaches, dizziness, trouble balancing, and drowsiness can all be seen in dehydration. Headaches, nausea, sensitivity to light and sensitivity to noise can be seen in patients with migraine headaches or athletes with a hangover, a not uncommon entity in college athletes. Patients who suffer from clinical depression often feel sad, with decreased energy. Doctors must therefore understand the circumstances that resulted in the athlete's symptoms, how the symptoms have changed since they started, and other medical problems the athlete has. All of these factors will help clinicians determine whether or not a given athlete has sustained a sport-related concussion.

Almost all assessments in medicine start with what is known as the history. The history refers to the patient's or athlete's description of how the injury occurred, how his or her symptoms started, and how the symptoms have changed since they started. After listening to patients describe their injuries and the symptoms that are bothering them, doctors often ask a series of questions to get more information. Some common questions asked by doctors to help them obtain further history are:

- When did the symptoms first start?
- Have they changed since you first noticed them?
- Are there certain things which make your symptoms worse?
- Are there certain things which make your symptoms better?
- Have you ever experienced symptoms like this before?
- Have your symptoms become worse since they first started?
- Have they become better since they first started?

By answering these questions as accurately as possible, athletes help their doctors determine whether or not it is likely they have sustained a concussion. Sometimes at the end of this question and answer session it is clear that the athlete has sustained a concussion. For example, let us suppose an athlete says to his doctor:

I was playing ice hockey a week ago. I felt great at the start of the game. I was in the best shape of my life. My team was playing for the number one spot in the division. I was behind my opponent's goal when I briefly lost control of the puck. As I was looking down at the ice, trying to regain control of the puck, I was struck by one of the opposing defensemen. I didn't see the blow coming. He lifted me off my skates. The back of my head struck the boards as I fell. My head bounced off the ice. The next thing I remember I was being helped off the ice by one of my teammates and the athletic trainer. They told me I had been knocked unconscious for a few seconds. I had a killer headache and felt a little woozy. After a few minutes I started throwing up. The athletic trainer was concerned. He put a brace on my neck and had the ambulance take me to the emergency department.

The doctor there ordered a CT of my brain which he told me was normal. He said I had a concussion and should stay out of hockey. And he told me to follow up here with you. Since then I've been feeling a lot better. I still get headaches almost every day but they are not half as bad as they were first few days after I got hurt. I still have a little bit of trouble sleeping. My girlfriend says I still seem a little bit out of it from time to time. But I feel a whole lot better than I did the first few days after injury.

In this example it is very clear that the athlete has sustained a sport-related concussion. He was feeling great at the start of the game, without any symptoms at all. He sustained a rapid blow to the body, followed by two blows to the head. He developed the immediate onset of headaches, nausea, confusion and other symptoms which have gradually been improving, but have not yet completely gone away. He has had a CT of his brain which was normal, letting the doctor know that there was no bleeding in the brain, bruising of the brain, swelling of the brain, or other injuries which are causing his symptoms.

Sometimes, as in the example above, it is easy to know whether or not an athlete sustained a concussion. However, at times, it can be more difficult. For example, suppose the athlete instead said to his doctor:

I had been sick for a few days before the game. A lot of the guys on the team felt sick. Some had vomiting. Others had diarrhea. Some had both. Still I felt good enough to play. As the game went on, I started to get a headache. I noticed I felt a little nauseous. At one point I skated over to the bench and told the athletic trainer I wasn't feeling well. He had me sit down and gave me some Gatorade. I threw up a couple of times and he became concerned. He thought maybe I had suffered a concussion. I don't remember taking any big hits or any hits to the head. But he said I got banged around a few times. Anyway, he wanted me to come see you to get checked out. I've been feeling better over the last few days but I still don't feel 100 percent back to normal. I feel a little out of it, at times. I think I just caught a stomach bug.

In this situation it is much more challenging to tell whether or not the athlete has sustained a sport-related concussion. Certainly, a concussion can cause an athlete to have headaches, feel nauseous, vomit, and feel "out of it." It could be that this athlete sustained a sport-related concussion and that this concussion is the cause of his symptoms. But the symptoms could also be due to a stomach virus. Indeed, many of the other players on this athlete's team have recently been suffering from what seems like a stomach virus. The athlete himself felt ill, even before the game started. It could be he came down with the same illness. Further complicating the picture, he may have come down with the same viral illness that his teammates had *AND* sustained a sport-related concussion. He may be suffering from both. In this case, it is much harder to tell whether or not the athlete has sustained a sport-related concussion. His doctor may perform further tests and assessments to help determine whether or not this athlete has been concussed.

Once it has been determined that an athlete has sustained a sport-related concussion, the athlete, the coaches, and the parents often ask what "grade" concussion the athlete has suffered. Similarly, when I hear news reports about professional athletes who sustain concussions, the reporter often refers to the grade of the concussion. Statements such as, "the cougars will be at a distinct disadvantage this weekend as their star quarterback is out injured after having suffered a grade 2 concussion," are common. However, those of us practicing sports medicine no longer grade concussions. The terminology is mostly still used due to historical reasons.

Historically, concussions were graded. A grade 1 concussion was thought to be milder than a grade 2. Grade 3 concussions were thought to be more significant than either grade 1 or grade 2. Several factors were used to determine the grade of a concussion. Athletes who lost consciousness at the time of their concussion received a higher grade than those that did not. Athletes who were knocked unconscious for longer periods of time received higher grades than those who were unconscious for shorter amounts of time. Athletes who suffered amnesia as part of their concussions were given a higher grade than those who did not; the longer the period of time for which the athlete had a loss of memory, the higher the grade of concussion. These grades were used to determine how long an athlete should be removed from sports after sustaining a sport-related concussion. This was a very convenient system for doctors and other clinicians managing sport-related concussions. Clinicians could simply look up the grade of an athlete's concussion, ask how many concussions the athlete had sustained previously, and use standard guidelines that specified how long the athlete should remain out of play before being returning to his or her sport. It turned out, however, that this approach was not the best for athletes. Some were held out of play, unnecessarily, even after full recovery. Others were put back to play too soon, prior to full recovery.

A NOTE ABOUT GRADING SYSTEMS: While grading systems have been abandoned in favor of more individualized management, they were extremely beneficial during their time. When the first grading systems were developed, few medical professionals took concussion seriously. Athletes were often sent straight back into play after sustaining a concussion, without another thought. These grading systems were instrumental in drawing much needed attention to the issue of concussive brain injury in sports. They allowed many athletes to recover from their injuries, prior to sustaining an additional concussion.

Grading systems were abandoned in the consensus and agreement statement from the first international conference on concussion in sports which was published in 1999. Those clinicians involved in the assessment and management of sport-related concussions had noticed that athletes who were knocked unconscious for brief periods of time often recovered more quickly than those who did not lose consciousness. Therefore, it seemed inaccurate to diagnose those who did not lose consciousness with a lower grade of concussion. Furthermore, grades were used to determine the period of time that an athlete was removed from sports. It did not make sense to keep those who recovered more quickly out of sports for longer periods of time than those who recovered more slowly. For this and for several other reasons, the use of grading systems was abandoned. Nowadays, when making decisions to return an athlete back to play after he or she has recovered from a sport-related concussion, doctors consider each case individually. Rather than simply looking up a standard guideline in a book, doctors take the whole clinical picture into consideration. Factors which may help determine the amount of time an athlete is asked to remain symptom free before returning to contact include:

- the length of time over which the athlete had symptoms from the concussion
- the length of time it took for the athlete to recover his or her brain function after the concussion
- the length of time it took the athlete to recover his or her balance after the concussion
- the amount of brain dysfunction associated with the athlete's concussion
- the intensity of symptoms suffered by the athlete after the concussion
- the number of concussions the athlete has sustained over his or her lifetime
- the amount of time that elapsed in between the athlete's concussions
- the amount of force that was required to produce concussive brain injury in the athlete
- whether or not the amount of force required to produce a concussion in the athlete has changed over time

All of these factors help determine the degree of injury sustained by the athlete. They help make decisions about how much recovery time is required for an individual athlete after a sport-related concussion. They factor into decisions about when to return an athlete to contact or collision sports. They also factor into decisions about whether or not an athlete should ever be returned to contact or collision sports.

In summary, a concussion is a traumatic injury of the brain. It results from a rapid, rotational acceleration or spinning of the brain. It is a functional injury to the brain, meaning that the brain is not able to work properly when it is concussed. However, a concussion does not result in significant bleeding, bruising, swelling, or other structural injuries to the brain. The brain cannot work properly after a concussion because the electrolytes that help the brain operate under normal circumstances have been disturbed. The severity of a concussion cannot be determined at the time of injury, but rather, is determined by assessing the factors which led to the injury in the first place, and monitoring the length of time required for the athlete to completely recover.

SUGGESTED READINGS

Aubry, M., et al., Summary and Agreement Statement of the First International Conference on Concussion in Sport, Vienna 2001. Recommendations for the Improvement of Safety and Health of Athletes Who May Suffer Concussive Injuries. *Br J Sports Med*, 2002. 36(1): 6–10.

Giza, C. C., and D. A. Hovda, The Neurometabolic Cascade of Concussion. *J Athl Train*, 2001. 36(3): 228–35.

Holbourn, A., Mechanics of Head Injury. *Lancet*, 1943. 2: 438–41.

Ommaya, A. K., and T. A. Gennarelli, Cerebral Concussion and Traumatic Unconsciousness. Correlation of Experimental and Clinical Observations of Blunt Head Injuries. *Brain*, 1974. 97(4): 633–54.

Shaw, N. A., The Neurophysiology of Concussion. *Prog Neurobiol*, 2002. 67(4): 281–344.

3

SPORT–RELATED CONCUSSION: HOW COMMON IS IT?

On October 27, 2007, the Philadelphia Flyers were playing the Boston Bruins. The score was 0 to 0 with 3:53 remaining in the first period. The puck was sent from just over the center line to behind the Flyers net. Boston Bruin Patrice Bergeron and Philadelphia Flyer Randy Jones skated after it. Bergeron arrived there first, sending the puck to his right, around the back of the net. Jones finished his body check on Bergeron, striking him from behind. Bergeron's face was thrown up against the edge of the dasher board. Jones' momentum carried him into Bergeron, compressing the Bruin's head into the boards further. Bergeron fell to the ice. He was motionless. He was unconscious.

Patrice Bergeron was concussed.

This case drew a great deal of media attention, particularly in the Boston area. It illustrated several poorly understood points about sport-related concussion. First of all, Patrice Bergeron missed the majority of the remaining hockey season due to his concussion. For many sports fans at the time, a concussion was thought to be a minor injury that might cause an athlete to miss, at most, one week of play. Furthermore, this concussion occurred during ice hockey. Certainly American football receives a larger share of the medical and sports media attention regarding sport-related concussions. Given the large number of athletes playing American football, more football players sustain sport-related concussions in any given year than the athletes of other team sports. However, as we shall see, several studies suggest that the proportion of ice hockey players sustaining a concussion over a given season is higher than that of the American football players.

This chapter will discuss many of the sports during which concussions occur. The relative frequency of concussion in each will be described. When known, various activities of the sport that increase the risk of concussion will be reviewed. Comparisons between male and female athletes playing the same sport will also be considered.

Sport-related concussion is a common injury. Exactly how common depends on the sport being played, the level of competition, the age of the athletes, etc. Furthermore, estimations are complicated by underreporting of the injury. Since a concussion cannot be "seen," athletes are able to conceal it from athletic trainers, team physicians, coaches, and parents. And many of them do. A 2004 study of high school American football players revealed that less than half of those sustaining a concussion reported it to anyone. Several reasons are given for this lack of reporting. Many younger athletes do not realize they have sustained a concussion. Fewer realize that a concussion is a traumatic brain injury. They believe they have merely "had their bell rung" or been "dinged." Even athletes who are knocked unconscious at the time of their injury often do not realize that they have sustained a concussion. In one medical study, high school athletes were allowed to write freely at the end of their questionnaires. One athlete recalled being sent to the athletic director after being knocked unconscious in order to see if he had a concussion. His interpretation after the meeting was that he did not have a concussion, despite the fact that he was knocked unconscious. He was free to return to sports. As athletes become older and more competitive, their reasons for underreporting change. Many become afraid that reporting the injury jeopardizes their chance to keep their position on the team. Many are afraid that if they report their concussion, it will jeopardize their chance to play at a higher level. Some are seeking a chance to play in college. College athletes may be trying to go professional. Either way, this underreporting makes accurate estimations of injury difficult.

Furthermore, how commonly an injury occurs can be measured in a variety of ways. It can be measured as the number of players who sustain a concussion during a season. However, this fails to account for athletes who receive minimal or no play time. Furthermore, the rates of concussion are higher during competition than they are during practice. Sports like American football have relatively few games per season when compared to basketball or ice hockey. Measuring the numbers of concussions occurring per season does not take into account the number of competitions per season. In addition, some athletes will sustain multiple concussions during a single season. Measuring only the percentage of athletes who sustain a concussion during a season does not take into account those who sustain multiple concussions. In order to address these inaccuracies, some investigators have measured the number of concussions occurring for every "athletic exposure," where each practice and each competition count as one "athletic exposure." Others measure how many athletes will sustain a concussion out of every 100,000 playing a given sport. Still others measure the percentage of total injuries during a season accounted for by concussions.

Studies have consistently demonstrated that, with the exception of cheerleading, concussions are more likely to occur during competition than during practice. This makes sense, as competitions are usually more intense and played more ferociously than practices. Taken all together, it is estimated that as many as 3.8 million sport-related traumatic brain injuries occur each year. The vast majority of these injuries are concussions.

Concussions account for 9 percent of all organized athletic injuries in U.S. high schools. In pediatric patients, 30 to 50 percent of all concussions seen in U.S. emergency departments occur during sports. In United States colleges, concussions represent 6 percent of all organized athletic injuries. Approximately 20 percent of concussions that involve a loss of consciousness occur during sports and recreation.

AMERICAN FOOTBALL

American football is a fast-moving, hard-hitting, exciting game, watched by millions of Americans each week. Given its popularity, it is one of the most frequently played sports by younger athletes. The recent retirement of some high-level professionals after sustaining multiple concussions has resulted in a lot of media attention about the rate of sport-related concussions in American football.

Approximately 1.8 million total athletes participate in American football annually, including, 1.5 million high school athletes. It is not surprising, given the large numbers of athletes participating in it, that American football accounts for the majority of the concussions that occur during team sports in the United States. In fact, some studies suggest that more than half of all sport-related concussions occurring in organized high school sports occur during football. Other studies suggest that 4 to 5 percent of high school and college football players will sustain a concussion during any season. However, many of these studies considered only those injuries diagnosed by the team's athletic trainer. As mentioned above, many athletes do not report their concussions. Interestingly, studies in which players have been asked directly and confidentially to report their symptoms after sustaining a blow to the head have revealed much higher rates of concussion, ranging from 15 to 45 percent of players per season.

Given the high rates of concussion in American football, in addition to the large number of athletes participating in it, efforts are being made to try to reduce the number of sport-related concussions that occur in American football. These efforts consist of rule changes, technical modifications to football helmets, changes in strength and conditioning, rule changes, and stricter, more consistent rule enforcement. These efforts have been inspired by former football players, or the loved ones of former football players, who have suffered the effects of multiple concussions. Many readers may know the story of Christopher Nowinski, a former college football player from Harvard University and former professional wrestler who was forced to retire after sustaining multiple concussions that led to long-term problems. He is the author of the book *Mind*

Games: The NFL's Concussion Crisis. I highly recommend this book to any athletes participating in high-risk collision sports such as American football.

ICE HOCKEY

Several studies suggest that ice hockey carries a higher risk of concussion than American football. Although this surprises many people, studies which directly compare the two sports show that concussions are more common in ice hockey than in American football. The percentage of ice hockey players who sustain a concussion in a given season is higher than the percentage of American football players who sustain a concussion in a given season. A medical review of concussion in contact and collision sports that included American football, ice hockey, rugby, and soccer revealed that, for high school male athletes, ice hockey had the highest rates of concussion.

BASEBALL AND SOFTBALL

Approximately 720,000 high school athletes compete in baseball and softball per year. Concussion accounts for 3 to 6 percent of all injuries occurring during baseball and softball. However, the way in which baseball players sustain concussions differs from that of softball players. In baseball, concussions most often occur when the player is struck in the head with the ball. Usually, the player is struck in the head with a pitch. In softball, however, while about half of concussions occur when the player is struck in the head with the ball, the remaining half are due to player-to-player collisions, collisions between a player and the outfield wall, or when the player's head strikes the ground after a fall.

BASKETBALL

Basketball is one of several sports that are popular with both boys and girls, men and women. As such, it gives us a unique insight into the effects gender might have on the rates of concussion. In girls' basketball, concussion accounts for 5 to 8 percent of all injuries, while in boys' basketball it accounts for about 4 percent of all injuries. Some studies have suggested that high school girls who play basketball have a higher risk of concussion than high school boys who play basketball.

SOCCER

Soccer is also popular among male and female athletes. Again, this dual popularity allows us to compare the rates of concussions between boys and girls who play soccer. Much like basketball, studies which compare the number of concussions that occur in girls' soccer to the number of concussions that occur in boys' soccer suggest that girls may be at higher risk.

Overall, head injuries account for somewhere between 4 and 20 percent of all injuries in soccer. The goalkeeper seems to be at an increased risk of concussion when compared to other players. However, as noted above, athletes are often reluctant to report their concussion, which makes estimations of the rates of concussion difficult.

Some authors have suggested that the rates of concussion in soccer are similar to those in American football. However, this seems unlikely. These results are often cited by those who are comparing one medical study conducted in soccer players to a separate medical study conducted in football players. However, such comparisons are ill advised. Medical studies that use the same methods and same populations to compare the number of concussions occurring in soccer, American football, and several other sports reveal that concussion is a much more common occurrence in American football than it is in soccer.

When discussing sport-related concussion, soccer deserves some extra attention. The sport of soccer is unique in that players use their heads to advance the ball, pass to their teammates, and shoot on goal. This has led to speculation that concussion in soccer occurs from purposeful heading of the ball. Some studies have revealed poorer brain function in former soccer players than the general population. In particular, soccer players who report that they used to head the ball more often than their teammates had poorer brain function later in life than those former players who reported they purposefully headed the ball less often. Such studies have further fueled the speculation that purposeful heading of the ball causes concussions.

However, several other studies refute such a conclusion. In one such study, soccer players had their brain function measured before and after a soccer practice, which included 20 minutes of a dedicated heading exercise. No changes in brain function were noted. Since concussion often results in a decrease in brain function, the authors conclude purposeful heading does not cause concussions. Other studies have documented all of the concussions that were sustained over the course of a soccer tournament. Investigators reviewed how the concussions occurred by watching videotapes of the games. In such studies, no concussions occurred as a result of purposeful heading of the ball. Thus, many people feel concussions do not occur as a result of purposeful heading.

Since opening the Sports Concussion Clinic in the Division of Sports Medicine at Children's Hospital Boston in November 2008, we have cared for nearly a thousand patients with concussions. Only a few have reported sustaining their concussions from purposeful heading of the ball. All of them were children.

Therefore, I believe that purposeful heading of the ball is unlikely to cause a sport-related concussion. If an adult or teenage athlete sees the ball coming, sets up, and appropriately heads the ball with proper technique, concussion is unlikely. However, I believe for children, it is possible to sustain a concussion from purposefully heading the ball. One can imagine a young child, perhaps new to soccer, who is still developing physical coordination, standing under a ball that was punted up high by the goal keeper, and delivering a poorly timed, uncoordinated blow. The ball may have more of an effect on the acceleration of the child's head than the child's head has on the acceleration of the ball. In this situation, I believe concussion is possible. The risk of this scenario is likely increased if children are sent out to play with adult-size soccer balls, as opposed to smaller balls more suitable for their size.

Some have suggested that perhaps children should not be allowed to head the ball until they reach a certain age and have become stronger and better coordinated. I believe, however, this would be a mistake. As children become stronger and better coordinated, they are able to kick the ball at a much greater velocity. It seems unwise to have their first time trying to head a ball occur at an age when the ball can be kicked with significant speed and force. Instead, using smaller, softer balls that weigh less while children are younger allows them to develop the skills necessary for proper heading of the ball. This seems like a safer approach. They can learn proper technique, develop strength, and master the timing and coordination necessary for proper heading of the ball when young, before they begin to play with an adult-size ball that can be kicked with significant force.

LACROSSE

First played by the Native Americans, lacrosse is a sport growing in popularity in the United States. For the reader unfamiliar with it, lacrosse has rules similar to ice hockey, but it is played on grass or turf. Players carry a stick with a net on the end of it. The net is used to carry the lacrosse ball. In order to score, the ball has to be thrown into the opponent's net, past the goalkeeper. Boys' and men's lacrosse are collision sports, where players are allowed to collide body to body, and defending players are allowed to use their sticks to strike at the offending player who is carrying the ball, in order to free it from his possession. According to the rules of women's lacrosse, such contact is not allowed.

Although fewer people play lacrosse than many other sports, concussion rates in lacrosse are fairly high. As in most collision sports, concussions in lacrosse most often occur during body-to-body collisions with an opponent. But they also occur from collisions with the ground, and from being struck in the head with the ball.

RUGBY

As with many collision sports, concussion is common in rugby, accounting for about 16 percent of all injuries. It usually occurs secondary to body-to-body contact with another player. In one study, concussions accounted for 40 percent of all injuries that occurred during illegal or foul play. Unlike soccer and basketball, the risk of concussion in women's rugby is similar to that in men's.

SKIING AND SNOWBOARDING

Downhill skiing and snowboarding are popular sports in which amateur participants travel at surprisingly high rates of speed, surrounded by snow, ice, trees, large metallic chair-lift poles, and fellow snow sport enthusiasts. Head injuries account for up to 20 percent of all injuries in these sports. Recently, some high-profile celebrities have sustained tragic head injuries, drawing much needed attention to the risks of these sports. When I was growing up in New England, the use of helmets while skiing was almost unheard of. Now, it is the norm.

In fact, I went skiing with a bunch of work colleagues several years ago. When we arrived at the ski slope we took all of our equipment from the car and headed for the bottom of the chair lifts. Once I had my skis attached and my poles ready, I looked up and saw that I was the only one, in a group of five or six skiers, who was not wearing a helmet. In addition to calling me crazy, they laughed and joked about how it was ironic that the physician among us whose career was dedicated to caring for athletes who sustain head injuries in sports was the only one without a helmet. Until that point, it had never occurred to me to wear a helmet while skiing. Now, I wouldn't go downhill skiing without one.

As men and women both participate in these downhill sports, comparisons can be made between the genders. Male skiers are nearly twice as likely to sustain a head injury than women skiers. Furthermore, concussions sustained by female skiers are more often due to collisions with another person, while those sustained by male skiers are more often a result of collisions with an object.

COMBAT SPORTS

Wrestling is a combat sport that does not allow for deliberate blows to the head by the opponent. Rather, combatants try to control one another by placing their opponents in various holds. Concussion accounts for 4 to 5 percent of all injuries in wrestling. Nearly half of the concussions in wrestling are due to takedowns.

Unlike wrestling, combat sports such as boxing, allow for purposeful blows to the head. Boxing is unique in that one of the main purposes of the competition is to concuss your opponent. If you deliver a blow to your opponent that knocks him unconscious for 10 seconds or longer, you win the bout. If you do not knock your opponent unconscious, but are able to concuss him such that he is dazed, confused, off balance, or has a slower reaction time, your task of delivering further blows becomes easier. It is this nature of boxing that has made it so controversial, especially when it comes to children participating. Without entering into the controversy, I will simply say that concussion is a common occurrence in boxing. Perhaps more concerning, the possible effects of multiple blows to the head that do not result in concussion have been raised recently. This will be discussed further in chapter 11.

Perhaps even more controversial than boxing is mixed martial arts, the popularity of whose competitions have risen dramatically over the last 20 years. Similar to boxing, mixed martial arts allows for blows to the head of one's opponent. Once again, the bout can be won by knocking the opponent unconscious, and significant advantage can be gained by concussing one's opponent, even if he is not knocked unconscious. Studies suggest that a concussion occurs in one out of every 10 mixed martial arts matches.

CHEERLEADING

Cheerleading has changed dramatically over the last 40 years. When I was a kid, cheerleaders literally led the cheers of the crowd. They organized and inspired the crowd. Occasionally, they might tumble, or do some handsprings. Nowadays, however, major cheerleading squads are more like a combination of gymnasts and acrobats. They perform stunts, often as high as 30 feet in the air, without the added precaution of pads or netting. They are thrown up in the air by other cheerleaders, and come crashing down into their colleagues' arms. Thus, it is not surprising that the rates of concussions occurring in cheerleaders have risen dramatically. Cheerleading has the unique distinction of being one of the only sports in which concussion is more common during practice than competition. As might be expected, more than 90 percent of concussions in cheerleading occur during stunts.

SHOULD CHILDREN PARTICIPATE IN THESE SPORTS?

In order to practice medicine, one must continuously weigh the potential risks of a given action against its known or potential benefits. One must weigh similar risks and benefits when encouraging children to participate in sports. While concussion is a risk in nearly all sports, the benefits from sports participation and athletic competition are innumerable. For children, sports participation increases their physical health, cardiovascular conditioning, strength, and endurance. It improves their self-image. It decreases the risk of obesity. By preparing for competition, children learn that they can improve their performance and skills through practice and hard work. Those children engaged in team sports learn to interact with their peers, to assist those who are less skilled, and to learn from those who are more highly skilled. They learn to cooperate. They learn to lead.

Furthermore, we in America are in the midst of an obesity epidemic. The rates of obesity in U.S. children have quadrupled in the last 30 years due, in part, to decreased levels of physical activity. The Centers for Disease Control and Prevention and the Surgeon General have issued recommendations aimed at decreasing obesity and increasing physical activity. Medical studies have shown that regular bouts of physical activity in childhood lead to more active lifestyles in adulthood.

For adults, sports participation increases strength, endurance, cardiovascular conditioning, mood, energy levels, and improves self-image. It lowers cholesterol levels. It decreases the risk of heart attack, stroke, obesity, depression. Exercise guarantees benefits. In fact, a person's individual, habitual amount of regular exercise is the most significant determinant of death from all causes. Most athletes will recover completely from their injuries. So, while we all should try to decrease the number of injuries sustained by athletes, and treat athletic injuries appropriately when they occur, athletes should be encouraged to continue to participate in sports. Even after sustaining a concussion, athletes should be encouraged to return to their preferred sports, as long as it is medically safe to do so.

In summary, concussion is a risk in almost any sport. Certainly combat and collision sports carry a higher risk of concussion than contact and noncontact sports. But the risks of concussion in contact sports, which do not involve purposeful collisions, are still significant. The risk of sustaining a sport-related concussion, however, is outweighed by the tremendous benefits that athletes derive from participation in sports. Concussions, if managed properly, should not prevent athletes from engaging in those sports that they love. For a very small minority of athletes who experience multiple concussions, or significant, prolonged, or incomplete recoveries from their concussions, sports participation may be restricted to certain safer activities.

Suggested Readings

Daneshvar, D. H., et al., The Epidemiology of Sport-Related Concussion. *Clin Sports Med,* 2011. 30(1): 1–17.

Fuller, C. W., A. Junge, and J. Dvorak, A Six Year Prospective Study of the Incidence and Causes of Head and Neck Injuries in International Football. *Br J Sports Med,* 2005. 39(Suppl 1): 3–9.

Gerberich, S. G., et al., Concussion Incidences and Severity in Secondary School Varsity Football Players. *Am J Public Health,* 1983. 73(12): 1370–75.

Koh, J. O., J. D. Cassidy, and E. J. Watkinson, Incidence of Concussion in Contact Sports: A Systematic Review of the Evidence. *Brain Inj,* 2003. 17(10): 901–17.

Nonfatal Traumatic Brain Injuries from Sports and Recreation Activities—United States, 2001–2005. *Morbidity and Mortality Weekly,* 2007. 56(29): 733–37.

Nowinski, C., *Head Games: Football's Concussion Crisis.* 2007, East Bridgewater, MA: The Drummond Publishing Group.

Shulz, M. R., et al., Incidence and Risk Factors for Concussion in High School Athletes, North Carolina, 1996–1999. *Am J Epidemiol,* 2004. 160: 937–44.

4

SPORTS EQUIPMENT: CAN HELMETS OR MOUTH GUARDS PREVENT CONCUSSION?

On October 3, 2010, the New York Giants dominated the Chicago Bears. The Giants defense seemed nearly unstoppable in the first half, tallying nine sacks of the Bears quarterback, Jay Cutler. On the second to last play of the half, Giants cornerback Aaron Ross, number 31, raced in unopposed from Cutler's left side. With the Bears quarterback secured within his grasp, Ross spun Cutler around 180 degrees and hurled him to the ground. The left side of Cutler's helmet, securely fastened to his head, bounced off of the ground sharply. Cutler was hesitant to get up. He was removed from the game.

Jay Cutler was concussed.

This chapter will discuss the potential role of personal protective gear in reducing the risk of concussions. The medical evidence regarding helmets, mouth guards, and other such protective equipment often advertized as capable of reducing concussion will be discussed.

Many people believe that football players wear helmets in order to reduce their risk of concussion. In fact, helmets were never designed for this purpose. Prior to the use of the modern-day helmets, catastrophic brain injuries, such as bleeding into the brain, skull fractures and massive swelling of the brain, used to occur at unacceptably high rates. Helmets were invented to reduce these catastrophic brain injuries, a task at which they are highly effective. But, it is likely that athletes wearing helmets play more aggressively than those without helmets. As a result, the introduction of helmets to a sport is more likely to increase the risk of concussion than to decrease it. Since helmets reduce the risk of death and devastating neurological outcomes after head injury, most people believe the potential for increased risk of concussion is a price worth paying.

Many companies advertise protective equipment by claiming it can reduce the risk of concussion. Companies selling helmets, mouth guards, headbands, "custom mandibular orthotics," and various other devices make such claims on their packaging, websites, and in advertisements. Yet the U.S. Centers for Disease Control, American Academy of Pediatrics, and experts on concussion in sports contend that there is no equipment available that has been proven to reduce the risk of concussion. As a result, many athletes, coaches, and parents are confused by the mixed messages. In the following pages I will discuss the reasons for the two separate messages and review the available medical evidence regarding these devices.

In the early 1900s American football was recognized as a dangerous sport. An offensive formation known as "the flying wedge" often led to significant injuries. In 1905, concerned by the number of deaths and catastrophic injuries sustained by American football players, President Theodore Roosevelt summoned college athletic directors to the White House for a meeting. This group of athletic leaders, led by New York University Chancellor Henry MacCracken, formed the group that ultimately grew to call itself the National Collegiate Athletic Association (NCAA). One of the main functions of the NCAA was, and remains to this day, to set the rules and regulations for intercollegiate American football and other sports.

However, it may surprise readers to know that football helmets were brought about by players, as opposed to rules set by the NCAA or other athletic organizations. Initially, the football helmet was nothing more than a leather hat and strap. The main intention was to prevent cauliflower ear, and perhaps to offer some protection to the head. Early versions of the modern-day plastic helmet did not appear until the 1930s. The helmet itself did not become mandatory in the National Football League until the 1940s. It may further surprise readers to learn that engineers designing the football helmet were not trying to prevent concussion. Back when the modern day football helmet was being designed, catastrophic injuries to the brain, such as swelling of the brain, bleeding into or around the brain, skull fractures, and death were much more common than they are today. The goal of these early helmets was to prevent such catastrophic injuries, which often resulted in death, coma, or neurological devastation. At the time, concussive brain injury was poorly understood. Most people, including physicians, did not recognize it as a significant injury. Therefore, there was no effort per se to try to prevent concussions, or to try to design helmets that could prevent concussion.

Only recently has the medical community realized that concussion results in true brain dysfunction. For this, and several other reasons discussed throughout this book, there is a renewed interest in trying to prevent concussions.

As stated above, some companies advertise protective equipment for reducing the risk of concussions. Yet many, if not most, medical experts maintain there is no such protective device available. This discrepancy likely results from differing interpretations of the available medical research data. We will review the available data here.

FOOTBALL HELMETS

As noted, football helmets were not originally designed to prevent concussions or even reduce the risk of concussion. They were designed to prevent catastrophic brain injury, death, or severe neurological injury. Despite that, there have been some studies examining the risk of concussions for athletes wearing various helmets. One such study suggested a slightly lower risk of concussion for athletes using a particular helmet. This led many to think that this helmet decreased the risk of sustaining a concussion while playing football. However, the methods and statistical analyses used to conduct this research left the conclusions vulnerable to doubt. Other studies have not been able to confirm these conclusions. Therefore, there is no convincing data demonstrating the ability of any given, available helmet to decrease an athlete's risk of concussion.

One additional medical study investigated the rates of concussion in athletes wearing more modern types of helmets, and compared them to the rates of concussion in athletes wearing older types of helmets constructed with earlier technology. Their results seemed to suggest that the newer helmet technology may reduce the risk of sport-related concussions, at least in American football. However, the study has been criticized for failing to account for all other possible factors. Those wearing the helmets with the newer technology were also wearing newer helmets. Those athletes wearing helmets made using older technology were wearing older helmets that had seen more playing time and thus suffered significantly more wear and tear. It could be that the perceived benefit was not, in fact, due to the new helmet technology but rather due to the fact that the helmets were new and therefore in peak condition.

Only in the last few years have engineers been designing helmets with the specific intention of reducing the risks of concussion. While this new effort is encouraging, at the time of this writing, there has been no published data on the effects of these newer helmet technologies. It is uncertain whether or not they will in fact reduce the risks of an athlete sustaining a concussion.

ICE HOCKEY HELMETS

The risks of head injury, cervical spine injury and concussion in ice hockey are high. These athletes are in a unique situation. They are on ice, a hard, slippery surface on which it is difficult to balance. They are wearing skates, which force them to balance their bodies on a thin, sleek, metallic blade. They are constantly colliding with one another in an attempt to knock each other off balance, off the puck, or out of the play. They are surrounded by hard dasher boards and Plexiglas. And they are capable of reaching high levels of speed, at times, exceeding 30 miles per hour. This is a setup for head and neck injuries. Thus, mandating the use of helmets in ice hockey is an obvious result. In order to reduce the risk of catastrophic head injuries, all ice hockey players should wear an undamaged, properly fitted helmet with the chin strap affixed appropriately.

Players, however, should know that these helmets will not reduce the risk of concussion. Playing with the head up, being aware of other players and objects around you, and being in peak physical condition are still the most effective defenses against sport-related concussions.

BICYCLE HELMETS

Perhaps the biggest impact helmets have made on athlete safety is in the realm of bicycling. Medical studies have demonstrated a decreased number of deaths in various populations since the introduction of bicycle helmet legislation. Unfortunately, for many of the same reasons discussed above in other sports, bicycle helmets do not definitively reduce the risk of concussion. In fact, some medical researchers feel that cyclists wearing bicycle helmets take more risks than those without helmets. Thus, while the risk of death and catastrophic brain injury may be decreased by wearing a helmet, the rates of concussion may in fact, increase. Either way, given their well-established ability to reduce death and catastrophic injury, cyclists should wear helmets.

I sold my car when my wife and I got married. Since then, I bike to work, to the store, to meet with friends, almost everywhere. I always wear my helmet. In addition, the employees of the Division of Sports Medicine at Children's Hospital Boston often have weekend bike rides together. I have never seen one of the members of our division cycling without a helmet.

SKIING AND SNOWBOARDING HELMETS

There is some evidence that helmets may reduce the risk of concussion in these alpine sports. There is good medical evidence that wearing helmets while skiing or snowboarding will reduce the risk of head injuries. A study involving over 20,000 skiers and snowboarders concluded that those wearing helmets had a 15 percent decreased risk of sustaining a head injury after a fall or collision compared to skiers and snowboarders not wearing a helmet. Please note, this study measured the risk of all head injuries, not specifically concussion.

Why helmets might help reduce the risk of concussion in one sport but not in others remains unclear. It could result from changes in behavior on the part of athletes. It is thought by some doctors and other medical researchers that in contact and collision sports such as football and ice hockey, there is a general respect for the head. Few, if any, athletes hope to cause harm or injure another athlete. Some have speculated that athletes who are not wearing helmets during these high-risk sports show some restraint when delivering a blow to one of their opponents' heads. However, when athletes are covered in helmets and other forms of padding, there may be a sense of indestructibility. Therefore, athletes who are playing fully padded are more likely to deliver and receive more aggressive and forceful blows than those who are not so effectively padded. Since, in general, the helmets and pads do not reduce the rotational acceleration of the head after impact, they have no effect on the risk of sport-related concussion. In skiing and snowboarding, however, concussion seldom results from a purposeful blow. Rather, concussive brain injury results from an accident in which the skier strikes a tree, the mountain, or other inanimate object. On occasion, it may occur from two skiers or snowboarders colliding. Since these injuries do not result from purposeful collisions, they're less likely to be affected by changes in behavior or attitude.

However, this is speculation. Other investigators have argued that, even in sports such as skiing or bicycling where purposeful blows are not delivered to one's opponents, wearing helmets increases the risk of concussive brain injury. These medical investigators hypothesize that athletes wearing helmets while participating in these sports engage in more risk-taking behavior. For example, they argue that cyclists wearing helmets travel at higher speeds, ride on more rugged terrain, dart in and out of traffic more readily, and are less likely to obey the rules of traffic. There is some medical evidence to support both sides of this argument. It seems likely, given the current available medical evidence, that modern-day helmets do not significantly decrease the risk of an athlete sustaining a sport-related concussion. In fact, they may increase the risk to some unknown degree.

IMPORTANT NOTE TO THE READER: While today's helmets may not be effective in preventing concussion, they are highly effective at preventing catastrophic brain injury. Therefore, all athletes participating in high-risk activities should wear a new, undamaged, properly fitted helmet.

Mouth Guards

Mouth guards have been cited by some as potentially preventing concussive brain injury. Several such studies were performed in cadavers. As readers of this book have already learned, the concussed brain is not structurally damaged; it is not significantly swollen, bruised, bleeding, or otherwise damaged. Concussion is a problem with brain function. The concussed brain does not work properly. Concussed patients have poor memory, poor concentration, headaches, difficulty sleeping, trouble with balance, etc. Since brain function cannot be assessed in a cadaver, we can draw minimal conclusions about the effects of preventing concussion from studies using cadavers.

Other studies have been performed in living athletes, both to determine whether or not concussions are less likely to occur in athletes wearing a mouth guard, or whether those wearing a mouth guard have fewer symptoms, less significant decreases in brain function, or faster recoveries.

In a study published in 2007 in the journal *Dental Traumatology*, Mihalik and colleagues measured neurocognitive function in two groups of athletes:

those who sustained a concussion while wearing a mouth guard and those who sustained a concussion while not wearing a mouth guard. They found no differences in brain function between the two groups—meaning that mouth guards did not prevent a loss of brain function after concussive brain injury.

In a 1987 study of rugby players published in the *British Journal of Sports Medicine*, Blignault and colleagues showed no statistical difference in the rates of concussion between rugby players wearing mouth guards and those not wearing mouth guards.

More recent studies have claimed that custom-made, form-fitting, special individualized mouth guards called custom mandibular orthotics (CMOs) may decrease the rates of concussion. However, the results are unclear. The methods used to conduct the research were poor, leading to unreliable and perhaps frankly erroneous conclusions. Therefore, no definitive conclusions can be drawn. Any effects of CMOs and other mouth guards on concussions remains unknown.

As with helmets, however, it is well established that mouth guards reduce the risk of facial bone fractures and dental injuries. Therefore, all athletes participating in sports that require the use of a mouth guard should wear an undamaged, properly fitting mouth guard while they are playing.

SOCCER HEADBANDS

Recently, soccer players, coaches and parents of soccer players have been asking about the ability of headbands to reduce the risk of concussion. Indeed, many headbands advertise such an ability. There is little medical evidence to support this assertion.

In a study published in the *British Journal of Sports Medicine* in 2000, McIntosh and McCrory studied eight commercially available head protectors designed for soccer players. They measured the ability of these protective devices to reduce energy at impact. They further investigated how well these devices maintained their function over time, after repeated impacts. As might be expected, they concluded that protective headgear for soccer players can reduce the risk of scalp lacerations, cuts, and abrasions, but that any reduction in the risk of sustaining a concussion is unlikely.

Other studies have suggested a potential benefit of soccer headgear in reducing the risk of concussion. So those of us caring for athletes cannot be certain as to whether or not these devices are effective. Certainly, medical studies showing a potential benefit, and those not showing a benefit, are limited. In some, there were other significant differences between the players wearing headgear and those not wearing headgear. In one study in particular, athletes who wore headgear were more likely to be female, to have suffered concussions previously, and to wear a mouth guard. Given these differences, these athletes may have played more cautiously than those not wearing headgear. It could be their cautious play that reduced their risk of concussion.

Or perhaps, given their history of previous concussions, this group was less likely to report their injury, for fear of losing play time. There are many possibilities that could explain the apparent association between headband use and decreased risk of concussion. Until further medical studies are conducted, no definitive conclusions regarding the use of soccer headbands to reduce the risk of concussion can be reached.

PLAYING SURFACE

Some investigators have suggested that the type of playing surface used by athletes may affect the rates of concussion or the severity of concussions. In a study published in 2002 in the *Journal of Trauma*, Rosanne Naunheim investigated the peak acceleration after impact on three different playing surfaces: natural grass, the indoor artificial turf of a practice field, and the indoor artificial turf in a domed stadium. Her results showed that peak acceleration was greatest with the indoor artificial turf of the domed stadium at 262 Gs, compared to 246 Gs for natural grass, and 184 Gs for artificial turf on the indoor practice field. These results suggest that the type of surface on which a game is played may affect the risk of sustaining a concussion after a fall to the ground.

In 2000, a study published by athletic trainer Kevin Guskiewicz examined the effect that playing surface had on immediate signs and symptoms of concussion. The results suggested that those athletes who sustained their concussions on artificial turf were more likely to lose consciousness than those athletes sustaining concussions on natural grass.

The data published thus far regarding playing surface and risk of concussion is preliminary. Furthermore, the type of surface on which athletes play is determined by many factors other than the risk of concussion. Expense, upkeep, space, location, and weather patterns all factor into a program's decision about which playing surface to use. Still, further research could clarify the effects of playing surface on concussion risk. Once clarified, programs could consider concussion risk as one of the factors used to help determine which playing surface they will employ.

Although some may find it discouraging, readers of this text can deduce an obvious explanation for the limitation in protective equipment in reducing concussion risk. For a moment, let us consider the way a shin guard works in soccer. When a soccer player without a shin guard is kicked by an opponent in the shin, a tremendous amount of force is delivered to the point on the shin struck by the toe box of his opponent's shoe. This blow to the shin causes significant pain, bruising, and occasionally fracture of the underlying shin bone. When the shin is covered by a shin guard, the amount of force delivered to the shin is the same. But rather than being delivered to one point on the shin, the force is now distributed over a larger surface area, specifically, the size of the shin guard. Thus, the force is absorbed by a larger area of the shin. This decreases pain, bruising, and overall injury.

Helmets operate in a similar way. Nearly the same amount of force strikes the player's head. But rather than the force being focused at the point of impact, it is distributed over the larger surface area of the helmet. We have already learned that concussion results from a rapid, rotational acceleration of the brain, or spinning, as a result of an impact. Helmets distribute the force of an impact over a wider surface area. But they do little to reduce the overall force. Therefore, they do little to reduce the resulting acceleration. Since it is the acceleration of the brain that causes the concussion, helmets can do little to reduce the risk of concussion. Newer technologies attempt to reduce the brain's acceleration after impact. Whether or not such technologies will be effective at reducing the risk of concussions in sports remains to be seen.

In summary, there is currently no reliable medical evidence showing that personal protective equipment reduces an athlete's risk of sustaining a sport-related concussion. Both scientific and medical investigations are under way to try to develop such personal protective devices. Hopefully, some effective equipment will be developed over the next decade or two. While they may not be proven to reduce the risk of concussion, however, helmets, mouth guards, and other personal protective devices are extremely effective at reducing the risk of catastrophic brain injuries, skull and facial bone fractures, dental injury, scalp lacerations, as well as many other injuries. Therefore all athletes participating in combat sports, collision sports, and contact sports should wear all appropriate protective equipment recommended by the sports' governing administrative bodies. In addition, all such personal protective equipment should be new, in proper working condition, and fitted appropriately.

SUGGESTED READINGS

Biasca, N., S. Wirth, and Y. Tegner, The Avoidability of Head and Neck Injuries in Ice Hockey: An Historical Review. *Br J Sports Med*, 2002. 36(6): 410–27.

Blignaut, J. B., I. L. Carstens, and C. J. Lombard, Injuries Sustained in Rugby by Wearers and Non-Wearers of Mouthguards. *Br J Sports Med*, 1987. 21(2): 5–7.

Danshevar, D. H., et al., Helmets and Mouth Guards: The Role of Personal Equipment in Preventing Sport-Related Concussions. *Clin Sports Med*, 2011. 30(1): 145–63.

McIntosh, A. S., and P. McCrory, Impact Energy Attenuation Performance of Football Headgear. *Br J Sports Med*, 2000. 34(5): 337–41.

Mihalik, J. P., et al., Effectiveness of Mouthguards in Reducing Neurocognitive Deficits Following Sports-Related Cerebral Concussion. *Dent Traumatol*, 2007. 23(1): 14–20.

Naunheim, R., et al., Does the Use of Artificial Turf Contribute to Head Injuries? *J Trauma*, 2002. 53(4): 691–94.

Theye, F., and K. A. Mueller, "Heads Up": Concussions in High School Sports. *Clin Med Res*, 2004. 2(3): 165–71.

5

New Medical Information: Why Is Concussion Taken So Seriously Nowadays?

Ted Johnson played linebacker for the New England Patriots. He was a hard-hitting, energetic, dynamic player, and a fan favorite. On August 10, 2002, during an exhibition game against the New York Giants, he sustained one of the many concussions that he suffered during his career. In a 2007 interview with *Boston Globe* reporter Jackie MacMullan, Johnson described the hit he delivered to Giant's running back, Sean Bennett, as "a terrific collision." It was a high-energy impact which resulted in Johnson being confused and blacking out.

Before the season had even started, Ted Johnson was concussed.

He was pulled from the game after discussing his injury with Patriots, medical staff. But several days later, despite suffering from persistent symptoms, he was pressured to return. He marks this as the start of his precipitous decline.

The remainder of his story is well known, having been described in several news articles, on several television shows, and featured on HBO's *Real Sports with Bryant Gumbel*. He reports suffering from crippling depression and apathy, often going days on end without shaving, showering, brushing his teeth, or leaving his apartment. He is, at times, unable to keep appointments. He and his physician, Dr. Robert Cantu, a world famous neurosurgeon and a leading expert in the management of concussive brain injuries, attribute Johnson's symptoms to the multiple concussions he sustained while playing football. And his symptoms are extensive, including, depression, fatigue, difficulty concentrating, poor memory and ringing in the ears, among others. While he told the *Boston Globe* he has only been diagnosed officially with three or four concussions, Johnson estimates he has suffered more than 30, adding, "I have been dinged so many times I've lost count."

This chapter will review the reasons why concussive brain injuries, and sport-related concussions in particular, are taken more seriously today than they were 25 years ago. Both medical and scientific studies will be reviewed.

There are four main reasons why concussion is taken much more seriously nowadays then it was 25 years ago.

1. Athletes who sustain one concussion are at a higher risk for getting another than athletes who have never had a concussion.
2. The effects of concussions are, to some extent, cumulative, meaning the more concussions athletes have, the worse their brain function becomes after each injury, and the longer it takes for them to recover from each concussion.
3. Some athletes who sustain concussions will develop problems later in life such as dementia, confusion, depression, and other problems. Some athletes with these problems have been diagnosed at autopsy with an entity now known as "chronic traumatic encephalopathy."
4. Athletes, particularly young male athletes, who return to sport before complete recovery from a concussion, are at risk for life-threatening swelling of the brain known as "second impact syndrome."

INCREASED RISK

Several studies have shown that athletes who have sustained one concussion are at increased risk for sustaining more. In 1977, a woman named Susan Gerberich investigated the number of concussions that occurred during high school football in Minnesota. She asked athletes to complete a questionnaire assessing details about their recent football season. She received responses from 3,063 players, representing 81 percent of those who received the questionnaire. Overall, approximately 19 percent of football players acknowledged sustaining a concussion during the 1977 fall football season. From her results, she noticed that the risk of being knocked unconscious was four times higher for those athletes who had been knocked unconscious before than for athletes who had never lost consciousness.

During the 1970s, there was still significant debate about how "concussion" should be defined. However, physicians on both sides of the debate agreed that an athlete who lost consciousness had sustained a concussion. Therefore, in order to avoid debate, it was often useful to separate out concussions that involved a loss of consciousness from those which did not involve a loss of consciousness. Certainly, these findings drew some much needed attention to the issue of concussive brain injury in American football. An athlete who had been knocked unconscious previously in his lifetime was four times more likely to be knocked unconscious during a given football season than an athlete who had never lost consciousness. This finding suggested that, perhaps, athletes who had sustained a concussion previously were more likely to sustain additional concussions.

During the late 1990s, a man named Mark Schulz collected data on nearly 16,000 athletes in North Carolina high schools and revealed a similar finding: those athletes who had sustained concussions in the past were twice as likely to sustain a concussion during the study period than those athletes who had never had a concussion. Several differences in the study by Schulz are worth noting. First of all, Schulz looked at all concussions, not only those that involved a loss of consciousness. Although some debate still existed in the late 1990s, it was more generally accepted that concussions occurred even when an athlete did not lose consciousness. Furthermore, Schulz looked not only at American football but other sports as well. This drew some much needed attention to the risk of concussive brain injury in sports other than American football.

Similar results have been seen in studies of college athletes. Kevin Guskiewicz, an athletic trainer from the University of North Carolina, followed nearly 3,000 college football players over the course of three seasons. His results showed that college football players with previous concussions were three times more likely to sustain a concussion than their teammates who had no previous concussions.

As these and other medical investigations revealed similar findings, the medical community realized that an athlete who has sustained a concussion at some point in his or her lifetime is at increased risk for sustaining sport-related concussions in the future when compared to athletes who have never had a concussion. The reasons for this increased risk are unknown. There are several possibilities.

A. It could be that some athletes are born with a predisposition or vulnerability to concussive brain injury. Perhaps the substance of their brain, the shape of their skull, or other physical characteristics make them more likely to sustain a concussion. When these athletes are included in medical studies, they are more likely to have sustained a concussion prior to the start of the medical study, since they are predisposed. Similarly, they are more likely to sustain a concussion during the medical study, simply because they are predisposed to concussive injury. Note, this increased risk has nothing to do with their prior injury. They are simply born predisposed to sustaining concussive brain injury. They have always been at higher risk.

B. It could be that it is simply a matter of playing time. Perhaps, athletes who receive more playing time sustain more concussions because they are more often at risk. The athlete on the ice playing hockey, or on the field playing football, is more likely to sustain an injury than the athlete on the bench, riding the pine.

C. It could be a matter of playing style. Perhaps athletes who sustain more concussions are too aggressive, constantly flinging themselves recklessly into risky situations. Perhaps when anticipating contact they often lead with their heads, placing themselves at greater risk of concussion. Or, maybe they are not aggressive enough. Maybe they are somewhat timid. As a result, a more aggressive player lines them up and delivers a well-timed, coordinated blow that not only renders them incapable of performing their competitive duties but also results in a concussion.

D. It may be a matter of body mass. Studies done in peewee and bantam ice hockey leagues have shown that athletes who are smaller in size are at increased risk for concussion compared to their larger counterparts. Perhaps smaller athletes sustain more concussions than larger athletes simply because they sustain more blows delivered by larger athletes capable of producing larger forces.

E. Finally, it could be that once athletes sustain a concussion, something changes in the brain that predisposes them to future concussions. This final possibility results in a great deal of concern for those of us engaged in athletics, sports medicine, and the management of concussive brain injury.

Currently, those of us in the medical field do not known which of these possibilities is true. It could be that all of the above explanations are true, each accounting for some proportion of repeat concussions in athletes. No matter the reason, athletes who have sustained one or more concussions are at increased risk for additional concussions. As a result, they should be managed closely with all available technologies.

CUMULATIVE EFFECTS

The effects of concussion are cumulative. There is some lasting effect on the brain after a concussion that persists, even after the athlete feels better. Athletes who sustain multiple concussions will have more significant symptoms, a more impressive decrease in their overall brain function, and will often take longer to recover than athletes who sustain only one concussion. Several medical studies have led to this conclusion.

As noted previously, a neuropsychologist is a clinician and scientist who has a doctoral degree in measuring brain function. In the 1970s, a neuropsychologist named Dorothy Gronwall measured the brain function of patients referred to her clinic after having sustained a concussion. She separated these patients into groups. One group consisted of patients who had sustained two concussions during their lifetime. The other group consisted of patients who had sustained only one concussion during their lifetime. She then measured the brain functions of the patients and compared their performance.

She found that those patients who were referred to her office after sustaining their second lifetime concussion had worse brain function than those who had sustained only one concussion. Furthermore, it took longer for the brain function of those who had sustained two lifetime concussions to return to normal than it did for patients who had sustained only one lifetime concussion. She concluded that the effects of concussion, therefore, are cumulative. These results suggested that there are some lasting effects on the brain after a concussion that do not resolve. At the very minimum, these effects make subsequent injuries more significant and more difficult to recover from.

Studies in athletes have shown similar findings. In the same study noted above by Kevin Guskiewicz, athletes took longer to recover from a concussion if they had sustained a previous concussion. Only 15 percent of players with one prior concussion had symptoms that lasted longer than a week. But for players who had three or more prior concussions, 30 percent had symptoms lasting longer than a week.

Even the events that occur at the time of injury may be different for athletes who have sustained multiple concussions, when compared to those who have sustained only one concussion. In a study performed by Micky Collins, a neuropsychologist at the University of Pittsburgh Medical Center, athletes who sustained a concussion were more likely to be knocked unconscious, to suffer confusion, and to suffer amnesia if they had sustained prior concussions.

It should be obvious to most readers that athletes are at constant risk for sustaining a concussion, particularly those involved in contact or collision sports. Therefore, athletes who sustain multiple concussions often sustain them within a relatively short time period. In fact, in the study by Kevin Guskiewicz, 90 percent of athletes who sustained repeat concussions during the same season suffered their concussive injuries within 10 days of one another. Furthermore, at the time these studies were conducted, many athletes were returned to sports before they were fully recovered from their concussions. This has led some to speculate that there is not, in fact, a cumulative effect of multiple concussive brain injuries when an athlete has proper time to recover in between each concussion. If an athlete has proper time to recover from one concussion before sustaining another concussion, some argue, there would be no measurable effects from the previous injury. The athlete would recover just as quickly as if he or she had only sustained one concussion. The deficits in brain function would be no different than if the athlete had only sustained one concussion. This leaves open the possibility that if athletes fully recover in between their concussions, they might not develop these cumulative effects. It is possible that recovering fully between injuries might minimize any potential, cumulative effects of injury. This hopeful possibility is one of the reasons why athletic trainers, doctors, and neuropsychologists recommend avoiding contact or collision sports until an athlete is completely recovered from a concussion.

It is interesting to note, however, that Dorothy Gronwall was not only studying athletes. Rather, she was studying all patients referred to her clinic with a concussion. Outside of sports, concussion is a relatively rare injury. It is uncommon for people who are not engaged in athletics to sustain a concussion. Certainly, having more than one concussion over the course of a lifetime is uncommon for non-athletes. Therefore, the length of time in between injuries tends to be greater for patients not playing sports than it is for patients playing sports. In Gronwall's study, the time in between concussions for those patients who had sustained two concussions ranged from five months to eight years. The average length of time in between the two concussions was 4.5 years. Therefore, statistically, it is likely that the majority of her patients, if not all of her patients, had recovered completely from the first injury at the time they sustained their second. Despite this, she was able to detect worse brain function and longer recovery times for those who sustained their second concussion. This suggests that there is, in fact, some cumulative, permanent effect on the brain after a concussion regardless of the amount of time an athlete or patient has to recover in between injuries.

While further research needs to be conducted into the potential effect of complete recovery in between injuries, most clinicians agree an athlete who completely recovers in between concussions is better off than the athlete who sustains an additional concussion before completely recovering from a prior concussion. Certainly, completely recovering from a concussion prior to sustaining an additional concussion decreases, if not completely eliminates, the risk of second impact syndrome, a catastrophic injury often leading to death, coma, or permanent loss of brain function, which will be discussed later in this chapter.

LONG-TERM EFFECTS

Many readers will remember classmates from their youth who spoke a little more slowly than others, seemed a little "spacey" or "out of it." When these students played sports like football or boxing, people used to say things like "that guy took too many hits to the head," or "that guy got his bell rung one time too many." The term punch drunk was fairly common. This may be a case, as often happens, where common sense and intuition precede medical knowledge. Although these remarks were often made jokingly, there was some understanding, some belief, that multiple blows to the head would result in problems with brain function, slowed thinking, slowed speaking, poor concentration, etc. Medical scientific studies are starting to confirm these previous suspicions.

Although the attention of the medical community has only recently been drawn to the long-term effects of concussive brain injury, one of the first medical articles to note the potential long-term effects of multiple blows to the head was published in 1928, in the *Journal of the American Medical Association*. In his article entitled "Punch Drunk," a physician named Harrison Martland detailed the physical characteristics of certain boxers described by fans as being "cuckoo, goofy, . . . slug nutty." The boxers Martland described developed an abnormal way of walking, where the men would drag a leg slightly behind them. Some would progress to develop more general slowing of all of their movements. Martland noticed these boxers had slowed speech, shaking of their hands, involuntary nodding of their heads. Some were unable to show expressions on their faces which became somewhat mask-like in their appearance. He reported that these men were often mistaken for being drunk. One such boxer was even excluded from a fight because he was suspected of being drunk at the time, when, in actuality, he was sober. Some of these pugilists became worse with time, losing the ability to think properly, to function in the world, to hold a job. Some were ultimately hospitalized in an asylum.

Martland observed that this disease was seen mostly in boxers who were known for their ability to take a punch. "Punch drunk" syndrome was uncommon in speedy, skilled, elusive fighters whose goal was to outbox their opponents by scoring more points, by landing more punches. Given their skill and agility, these types of boxers sustained relatively few square punches to the head. Rather, the illness Martland described was seen in boxers of the "slugging type," men who endured considerable blows to the head but managed to stay on their feet, engaged in the fight, seeking to land one giant knockout blow in order to win.

Those of you unfamiliar with boxing but who have seen the movies *Rocky* or *Rocky 2,* can still appreciate these two separate styles of boxing. Apollo Creed would be the skilled, agile, elusive fighter. His ultimate goal is to outbox Rocky Balboa. Creed is constantly bobbing and weaving, dodging the slow yet forceful punches of Balboa. Creed rarely sustains a square punch to the head. Rocky Balboa, on the other hand, is a boxer of the "slugging type." He is not as fast, skilled, or agile as Creed. He cannot possibly hope to outbox Apollo Creed. But given his enormous strength and power, he seeks to win the bout by delivering one, powerful, fatal knockout blow that knocks Creed unconscious for 10 seconds. Balboa endures considerable punishment, sustaining multiple blows to the head and body, yet remains on his feet in the hopes of delivering that one, mighty, winning blow. Balboa can take a punch. It is in this type of fighter, "the slugger," represented by Balboa, in which Martland described the entity he called "punch drunk."

The characteristics of "punch drunk" as described by Martland are remarkably similar to those described more recently in professional football players ultimately diagnosed with "chronic traumatic encephalopathy." This entity will be discussed further in chapter 11.

However, full-blown "punch drunk" syndrome or chronic traumatic encephalopathy is not the only effect of multiple blows to the head, or multiple concussions. A well-known study by athletic trainer Kevin Guskiewicz examined the proportion of retired American football players with impaired brain function later in life. He found that players who had sustained concussions were three times more likely to report problems with memory than those who did not sustain concussions. Furthermore, his results showed that the rates of brain dysfunction in retired football players who sustained three or more concussions during their career were five times higher than retired football players who did not sustain a concussion during their career. Those retired football players who had developed Alzheimer's disease did so at a younger age than the general American male population.

While this is concerning for long-term effects of concussions, there have also been studies that did not detect any long-term effects from sport-related concussions. As a result, there is ongoing controversy about whether or not concussions result in any long term problems.

There is little doubt in my mind that some athletes, as a result of multiple concussive brain injuries, lose some brain function that they never recover.

I am equally convinced, however, that many athletes who sustain sport-related concussions make full and complete recoveries, regaining all of their previous brain function. The differences between these two groups of athletes are unclear at this time. There are several possibilities:

1. Those who have lost some brain function may have sustained many more concussions than those who have retained their brain function.
2. Those who have lost brain function may have sustained injuries that involved greater forces than those who have retained their cognitive function.
3. Some people may be more vulnerable to the effects of concussion, such that they have a more difficult time recovering their brain function after a concussion, or after multiple concussions. This vulnerability may be due to their genetics, the shape of their brain, the shape of their skull, or other biological factors.
4. Those who have lost some brain function may have sustained repeated injuries without recovering fully in between each of them, while those who retain their brain function recovered fully in between their concussions.
5. There may be a certain age at which sustaining concussions results in a loss of brain function that is not recoverable, while athletes at different ages at the time of their concussions are able to fully recover.

One of the jobs of physicians, scientists, neuropsychologists, athletic trainers, and others involved in the care of athletes is to discover the reasons why certain athletes lose some of the capabilities of their brain as a result of sustaining concussions, while other do not. Such insights might lead to prevention and treatment strategies.

SECOND IMPACT SYNDROME

Although rare, second impact syndrome is tragic.

In 1984, two physicians named Saunders and Harbaugh described the tragic case of a man who died after sustaining a head injury. He was a 19-year-old college student and football player. He had been in a fistfight during which he received a blow to the head that knocked him unconscious. The day after the fistfight, he was taken to the school infirmary, where he had headaches and nausea. He was removed from football. Three days later he reported feeling better but still had a mild headache. He returned to football. During a play in which no one recalls any significant trauma to the head, or other major blow to the body, the patient became ill. He walked off the field and collapsed. He was taken to an emergency department, where he was noted to be unconscious. A breathing tube was inserted so that doctors could help maintain his breathing. A picture of his brain called a computed tomography (CT), or "cat scan," was taken. It showed significant swelling of the brain and a small amount of blood. He died several days later, despite medical and surgical treatments. Saunders and Harbaugh hypothesized that because this young man had not fully recovered from his prior concussion, that he had sustained during the fistfight, he was more susceptible to the catastrophic swelling of the brain that resulted from a blow so minor that none of his teammates could recall it.

Since that time, there have been multiple similar cases described in the medical literature. This occurrence has become known as second impact syndrome.

An athlete who is recovering from a concussion, but is not yet fully recovered, is at risk for second impact syndrome. When athletes return to play before they are fully recovered from a concussion, a second blow to the head, even a mild one, or even a blow to the body that results in a rapid movement of the head, can cause massive swelling in the brain. Since the brain is contained in the rigid bone of the skull, this swelling causes compression of the brain. In severe cases, the brain is squeezed through small holes within the skull. This squeezing of the brain through these small holes is known as "herniation." Herniation can lead to decreased blood flow to the brain, and ultimately to the athlete's death.

Every year during football season, there is an article in the newspaper about an athlete who returned to football before he had recovered completely from a concussion. Often, the athlete told his doctor, athletic trainer, and coach that he was better but confided to friends and teammates that he still had some lingering symptoms, such as headaches or nausea. And, although no one remembers any major blows to the head or collisions, the athlete develops massive brain swelling and dies.

Although second impact syndrome is rare, it has a devastating effect on those involved. Those who do survive second impact syndrome are neurologically devastated. They often spend many weeks to months in a coma. Many times they have a hole cut in their neck through which a permanent breathing tube is inserted. They are hooked up to a machine to help them breathe. They receive all of their nutrition intravenously as they are not awake enough or alert enough to eat or drink. The athletic trainer, team physician, primary care physician, and other medical personnel are left wondering about their relationship with the athlete. Often times they are confused as to why the athlete would not have spoken of his symptoms. They question whether or not there were other steps they could have taken in order to prevent the injury. They start to fear that other athletes on the team are perhaps downplaying their symptoms in order to return to play and are therefore at risk for second impact syndrome. They are often reluctant to allow future athletes to return after sustaining a sport-related concussion. Often the coaching staff suffers many of the same emotions. They too are left wondering whether their coaching had something to do with the athlete downplaying his symptoms. They wonder whether or not there was anything they could have done to prevent the injury. They worry about the remainder of athletes under their supervision. Second impact syndrome is perhaps hardest on the teammates of the injured player. While some of them may have been aware that the athlete was still experiencing symptoms from his concussion, most were unaware that returning to play prior to complete recovery from a concussion could lead to such a devastating outcome. They often feel a sense of guilt about not informing the athletic trainer, parents, or coaching staff that the athlete was still experiencing symptoms. They are devastated by the loss of their friend. They are haunted by thoughts that perhaps they could have prevented the injury. They fear for their own safety on the playing field.

Avoiding second impact syndrome is one of the main reasons why physicians, athletic trainers, neuropsychologists, and other medical professionals do not return athletes to sports until their symptoms have completely resolved.

Something else is worth noting about the case described by Saunders and Harbaugh. The athlete sustained his concussion in a fistfight, outside of organized athletic activity. While those of us in sports medicine concentrate on concussions that occur in sports, many athletes will sustain concussions outside of organized, supervised athletics. Given the lack of parental or medical supervision during these instances, diagnosing these concussions is even more difficult, especially without the help of the athlete. These circumstances should not be overlooked. Furthermore, when an athlete reports a concussion that was sustained outside of athletics, those of us involved in sports medicine are often still the best equipped to manage the injury.

Thus far, second impact syndrome has only been described in boys and young men. Perhaps there is something different about the male brain, or more specifically the young male brain, which predisposes it to second impact syndrome. It could be that male athletes are susceptible to this injury, whereas female athletes are not. I suspect, however, that girls, women and older men are equally susceptible and cases may be seen in the future. Since the majority of athletes playing contact and collision sports are young men and boys, and since second impact syndrome is rare, it is statistically more likely to occur in young male athletes. But the overall numbers of female athletes participating in contact and collision sports is increasing every year. It is possible that a case of second impact syndrome will occur in a female athlete in the future.

In summary, those who sustain one concussion are at increased risk of future concussions than those who have never suffered a concussion. The effects of multiple concussions are likely cumulative. For some athletes, there are long-term effects from sustaining multiple concussions. Second impact syndrome is a risk when athletes who are not completely recovered from a concussion are returned to sports. It often leads to devastating consequences.

SUGGESTED READINGS

Collins, M. W., et al., Relationship between Concussion and Neuropsychological Performance in College Football Players. *JAMA*, 1999. 282(10): 964–70.

Gerberich, S. G., et al., Concussion Incidences and Severity in Secondary School Varsity Football Players. *Am J Public Health*, 1983. 73(12): 1370–75.

Guskiewicz, K. M., et al., Cumulative Effects Associated with Recurrent Concussion in Collegiate Football Players: The NCAA Concussion Study. *JAMA*, 2003. 290(19): 2549–55.

Martland, H., Punch Drunk. *JAMA*, 1928. 91(15): 1103–7.

Saunders, R. L., and R. E. Harbaugh, The Second Impact in Catastrophic Contact-Sports Head Trauma. *JAMA*, 1984. 252(4): 538–39.

6

"Neuropsychological" or "Neurocognitive" Testing: What Is It and Should My Athlete Have It?

On September 26, 2009, the Florida Gators were beating the Kentucky Wildcats by a score of 31 to 7. It was the third quarter. The Gators star quarterback, Tim Tebow, called for the snap. He was looking to his right, when, from his blind side, he was drilled by Kentucky's number 94, Tyler Wyndham, who charged, unblocked, from the line of scrimmage. Wyndham's helmet struck Tebow's face-mask, rocketing his head backward. As he was pinned to the ground, his head bounced forward off of the leg of his teammate, Marcus Gilbert. As he lay on the field, he flinched once or twice, but was mostly motionless. It was several minutes before Tebow could be removed from the field. On the sidelines, he started to vomit. He was taken to a nearby hospital where he had a CT of the brain that was negative for bleeding. He was admitted overnight.

Tim Tebow was concussed.

The media coverage that followed was uncommon. Perhaps because of Tebow's stature and fame, his concussion received more media coverage than most. There was some good that came out of the coverage. Many younger athletes saw that Tebow was taken out of the game. Many sports fans unfamiliar with concussion management read about Tebow's "baseline" test and how he would retake it later, when doctors felt he was improving, to help assess when he was recovered. For many, this was the first they had ever heard of neuropsychological testing.

The terms neuropsychological testing and neurocognitive testing are often used interchangeably. When discussed in the context of athletes sustaining sport-related concussions, these terms mostly refer to computerized neuro-psychological testing.

Neuropsychology is a long-standing profession dating back to the earliest times of research in brain function. It is a subspecialty of psychology that deals with the function of the brain and how it relates to behavior. Neuropsychologists are clinician-scientists who assess brain functioning. They use standard tests to determine patients' cognitive, social, emotional, and behavioral functioning. They measure patients' reaction time and the speed with which patients solve problems. They assess patients' decisions, decision making abilities and the strategies patients use to make decisions. The data obtained during these observations and tests allow neuropsychologists to understand how a patient's brain is working. These measurements of brain function can be used to help determine appropriate treatments and interventions, clarify diagnoses, and assess relative strengths and weaknesses in many conditions such as attention deficit/hyperactivity disorder, learning disabilities, autism, Alzheimer's disease, and epilepsy (recurrent seizures). They can be used to assess brain function after injuries such as stroke, drowning, and traumatic brain injuries. In the setting of sports, they are most often used to measure brain function before and after a sport-related concussion.

In the 1980s, a group of neuropsychologists suggested measuring brain function in athletes who played American football. Given the large number of athletes playing American football, and the relatively high occurrence of concussions in American football, it seemed logical. Since that time there have been numerous medical studies investigating the use of neuropsychological testing in assessing sport-related concussions.

In 1999, a landmark study was published in the *Journal of the American Medical Association (JAMA)*. In this study, a neuropsychologist named Micky Collins, and his colleagues at the University of Pittsburgh Medical Center measured the brain function of 393 college football players prior to the start of a football season. Those athletes who sustained a concussion during the season were retested after their injuries. The results were remarkable.

Prior to the start of the season, those athletes who had sustained a concussion at some point during their life, performed worse on neuropsychological tests then those athletes who had never sustained a concussion. This has led some to suggest that the effects of concussion are permanent and do not resolve with time. But this cannot be concluded from these data. It is possible that the iower brain functioning measured by the tests was present before the injuries, and perhaps predisposed these athletes to sustaining a concussion rather than resulted from their previous concussions. Indeed, it is not hard to imagine that athletes with slower reaction times might be at increased risk for a sport-related concussion. Similarly, however, we can just as easily imagine that multiple concussions themselves led to permanently slower reaction times. Other studies, discussed later in this book, have been performed to address this question. The study by Dr. Collins and his colleagues showed convincingly, however, that concussion results in abnormal brain function after injury. Players performed worse on measurements of their brain function days after a concussion, than they did before the start of the season, when they were uninjured. This was remarkable because, at the time of this study, it was not commonly accepted that measurable brain dysfunction resulted from a concussion.

This study required an enormous amount of work. The neuropsychological tests took 30 minutes or more to perform for each athlete. They tested nearly 400 football players. So, while the results were revealing, it did not seem like a practical way to assess or monitor sport-related concussions. Many college football teams have 70–100 players. Testing each of them before the start of the season would require one or more trained neuropsychologists to spend 35–50 hours examining the athletes. A written report would have to be generated for each athlete. After each concussion, the tests would have to be repeated, often multiple times, while monitoring recovery. The team would have to pay for each test. Routinely allotting this amount of time in an already packed athletic training schedule would be difficult. While professional and some major college athletic programs might have the funding for such an endeavor, few, if any, high schools would. Furthermore, concussion occurs in other sports besides American football. The thought of performing these traditional neuropsychological assessments on every at-risk athlete at the beginning of each season, and again, often multiple times, after each concussive injury, seemed daunting. Indeed, it was unlikely to happen on a large scale.

The constraints of traditional neuropsychological testing led to the invention of computerized neuropsychological tests. These tests use a computer to measure brain function in place of some of the previous versions of traditional neuropsychological tests. Computerized versions have several advantages over the traditional testing paradigms. They allow for multiple preseason or "baseline" tests to be performed simultaneously. If there are enough computers available, the entire team can be tested at once. Since they are limited in their scope, medical personnel such as team physicians and certified athletic trainers can be taught to administer and perform limited interpretations of the tests. Computerized tests are more affordable than traditional tests. And they are more precise in certain areas of testing. For example, the computerized tests can measure an athlete's reaction time to one-thousandth of a second, much more precisely than a person with a stopwatch can measure.

While taking computerized neuropsychological tests, athletes are asked to complete several tasks. Often, they are given a series of words to remember. Periodically throughout the duration of the test, the athlete is asked to recall whether or not various words were a part of the original list. A similar list of designs or shapes is also presented, and athletes are asked periodically to recall whether or not various shapes were a part of the original list. There are tasks of memory and concentration, similar in many ways to the card game "concentration" that many readers will have played during their childhood, where athletes are asked to remember the location of various objects after they have been covered. There are tests dealing with numbers, letters, and various designs. Measurements are recorded of the number of tasks performed correctly, the number performed incorrectly, and the time it takes for athletes to complete each task. From these measurements, clinicians can obtain a quantitative measurement of the athlete's cognitive abilities. This is stored in the medical record.

Ideally, the athletes on teams engaging in sports with a significant risk of concussion will each undergo a baseline computerized neuropsychological test prior to the start of the season. This will be considered a measurement of their normal brain function, the functioning that their brain is capable of when it is not injured. Then, if an athlete sustains a concussion during the season, the test is repeated. This allows doctors, athletic trainers, and neuropsychologists to see how far the athlete's function has decreased. Furthermore, the test can be repeated to monitor recovery. Medical personnel can see how long it takes for the athlete to regain his or her preseason functioning.

While computerized neuropsychological tests are valuable in assessing and managing sport-related concussions, they should not be viewed as a replacement for traditional neuropsychological testing. In traditional testing, a trained neuropsychologist is able to detect aspects of brain functioning by observing how a patient approaches certain problems, handles difficulties, and processes information. During traditional testing, the neuropsychologist can interact with the patient to gain an understanding of how the patient handles a given task. This direct observation and interaction is lost with computerized testing. In addition, these tests are currently used mostly for the detection, assessment, and management of traumatic brain injury. Their potential role in identifying other disease processes and supporting other diagnoses is not yet clear. Finally, their interpretation is limited by the training and experience of the clinician using them. Physicians and athletic trainers can be taught to administer and interpret these tests to some extent. They can administer baseline tests and determine the validity of baseline tests. They can be taught to detect variations from baseline performance after injury and return to baseline performance during recovery from concussion. They can even be trained to detect some of the more common mistakes and misinterpretations of the directions by athletes, and learn how to correct for those mistakes by mathematically adjusting the patient's scores. However, there is no doubt that a trained neuropsychologist who has significant training and experience using computerized neuropsychological testing will be able to glean much more information from these tests. Such neuropsychologists are better equipped to interpret tests complicated by learning disabilities, attention deficit hyperactivity disorder, and other factors which effect computerized neuropsychological test scores. Ideally, all concussion action plans will include the services of a neuropsychologist with specific training in the administration and interpretation of computerized neuropsychological tests.

Similarly, neuropsychologists who are familiar with traditional test paradigms but have not trained on computerized tests will be limited in their ability to interpret the computerized test scores. As these tests are relatively new, there will be many practicing neuropsychologists who are not familiar with them.

For those who know how to properly administer and interpret these tests, they are highly valuable. Multiple medical studies have shown that these studies can help diagnose sport-related concussions and monitor recovery. Perhaps their most valuable quality is their ability to detect decreased brain function even after athletes report being symptom-free. Medical studies suggest that up to 30 percent of athletes who feel recovered from their sport-related concussions and report that they are symptom-free still have measurable deficits in their brain function for several additional days.

Prior to the routine use of neuropsychological testing in athletes at risk for sport-related concussions, athletic trainers and physicians managed these patients according to their symptoms. When athletes sustained a suspected concussion and told their team medical personnel about it, complaining of headaches, nausea, poor concentration, and other symptoms of concussion, they were removed from play. Once they informed the team's medical personnel that their symptoms had resolved, they were cleared to start the return to sports. This left players vulnerable to three potential issues. First, many athletes do not recognize their symptoms as indicative of a concussion. Second, as discussed earlier, many athletes, for various reasons, report being symptom-free despite remaining symptomatic. Third, medical personnel had no way of knowing which athletes had persistent brain dysfunction, even after they reported being symptom-free. Computerized neuropsychological testing can help resolve each of these issues, to some extent.

A study from the same group of investigators at the University of Pittsburgh used computerized neuropsychological testing to assess the brain function of athletes prior to the start of the season, in what is now known as a "baseline" test, and after a concussion occurred, in what is now known as a "post-injury" test. Their study revealed that nearly 19 percent of athletes who reported having no residual symptoms after a sport-related concussion still had abnormal neuropsychological test scores. These findings are significant. They show that athletes who report being symptom-free have not always recovered their full brain function. Incorporating computerized neuropsychological testing into a full concussion management program allows sports medicine clinicians to detect those athletes who, despite reporting full resolution of their symptoms, are still concussed.

A few points should be noted about neuropsychological testing in the assessment and management of sport-related concussion. First, it is only one of several tools clinicians use when managing an athlete who has sustained a concussion. The assessment of sport-related concussions should also include: a thorough medical history detailing how the injury occurred and the details of previous concussions; a thorough neurological physical examination to assess for other associated injuries; a thorough and honest symptom inventory; and a standardized balance assessment. Limiting the assessment to only one or two of these components of concussion assessment denies athletes the safest and best medical care.

Too often, I hear news reporters saying an athlete is "taking a concussion test" to see if he can return to his given sport. This is a misleading statement. Athletes who perform well on these neuropsychological tests, even those who reachieve their baseline scores, will often require further recovery time. An athlete who is still experiencing symptoms, for example, will require further recovery time. Athletes who still have poor balance as compared to their preseason balance will require further recovery time. Athletes who have been out of training for several weeks or months due to their injury will need to regain their former strength, agility, speed, timing, and coordination before returning to their activity. Finally, athletes who have sustained multiple concussions, severe symptoms after their concussions, significant cognitive dysfunction after their concussions, or prolonged recovery times will often require further time out of contact, even after their cognitive function has returned to baseline.

There is some debate as to when post-injury tests should be performed. If the test is being used solely to decide whether or not an athlete should be returned to play, then there is little point in conducting the test before the athlete's symptoms have completely resolved and his or her balance has been restored to its baseline level. Those athletes who still have poor balance or still have concussion symptoms will not be returned to sports no matter how well they perform on their neuropsychological tests. Thus, some clinicians will only perform these assessments when an athlete's symptoms have resolved and balance has been recovered. However, the tests may have other uses. For example, student athletes will have homework, quizzes, tests, term papers, and other academic assignments during their recovery. Thus, when deciding how much schoolwork they should undertake, and which academic accommodations should be put into place, computerized neuropsychological tests can be helpful. They may be performed prior to symptom resolution and balance recovery under these circumstances. In some cases, where schools are reluctant to put academic accommodations in place, these tests can serve as objective, quantitative evidence that the athletes are suffering from cognitive dysfunction. This will often help to convince schools of the need for accommodations during the recovery period.

Nearly all athletes should have baseline neuropsychological testing performed, prior to the start of the season. When we first started the Sports Concussion Clinic in the Division of Sports Medicine at Children's Hospital Boston, it never occurred to me the type of athletes we would be seeing. Certainly, I expected to see athletes playing football, ice hockey, rugby, lacrosse, soccer, basketball, and baseball. But I didn't fully realize how many patients I would see who sustained their injuries cycling, horseback riding, skiing, snowboarding, figure skating, and cheerleading. And it would never have occurred to me that I would see athletes who had sustained their concussions from swimming, dancing, rowing crew, and sailing. The more I practice medicine, the more I realize concussion occurs in all sports. Therefore, I would recommend any athlete to seek baseline computerized neuropsychological testing.

Certainly, some sports carry a higher risk of concussion than others. I would strongly recommend baseline computerized neuropsychological testing for all athletes engaged in collision and combat sports. Collision sports, as discussed in chapter 1 are those sports in which the delivery of blows to the body is a purposeful part of the sport. Common examples of collision sports are:

American football
men's ice hockey
men's lacrosse
rugby

Combat sports are those in which to athletes are engaged in a fight, albeit with specific rules and guidelines, supervised by a referee. Common examples of combat sports are:

boxing
mixed martial arts
karate
judo
wrestling

Furthermore, I would strongly recommend baseline testing for contact sports. Contact sports can be divided into two categories. Those in which contact occurs accidentally, meaning it is not a part of the activity, and those in which contact occurs incidentally, meaning it is a known, accepted part of the game but purposeful blows are not delivered. Common examples of sports in which contact is possible but is rare and accidental are:

skiing/snowboarding
horseback riding
pole vaulting
sailing
skateboarding
bicycling
gymnastics
cheerleading
springboard diving

Common examples of contact sports in which contact is an incidental but expected and accepted part of the game are:

soccer
baseball/softball
basketball

water polo
women's lacrosse
women's ice hockey
field hockey

In addition, I strongly recommend that all athletes who have sustained *one* concussion at some point during their lifetime undergo baseline computerized neuropsychological testing after they are recovered and before they return to sports of any kind. As already discussed in this book, athletes who have sustained one concussion are at increased risk for another. It would be unfortunate if these high-risk individuals were not managed with the best possible available means. Therefore, if possible, any athlete who has suffered one concussion should undergo computerized neuropsychological baseline assessment after he or she has recovered, before being cleared for participation in further sports activity.

In summary, neuropsychological testing is used to assess an athlete's brain function both before and after injury. It is one of several tools used to diagnose a concussion, monitor recovery from a concussion, and safely return an athlete to play after a sport-related concussion. Computerized neuropsychological tests are accurate, convenient, and represent a huge advancement in the management of sport-related concussions. They enable sports medicine clinicians to detect additional persistent concussions that may have been otherwise miscategorized as recovered. They are one of several tools used to assess and monitor recovery after a sport-related concussion. Most, if not all, athletes should undergo baseline neuropsychological testing. Athletes in high-risk sports and athletes who have sustained previous sport-related concussions should strongly consider having baseline neuropsychological testing performed.

SUGGESTED READINGS

Alves, W. M., R. W. Rimel, and W. E. Nelson, University of Virginia Prospective Study of Football-Induced Minor Head Injury: Status Report. *Clin Sports Med*, 1987. 6(1): 211–18.

Collins, M. W., et al., Relationship between Concussion and Neuropsychological Performance in College Football Players. *JAMA*, 1999. 282(10): 964–70.

Echemendia, R. J., *Sports Neuropsychology: Assessment and Management of Traumatic Brain Injury.* 2006, New York: The Guilford Press.

Erlanger, D., et al., Development and Validation of a Web-Based Neuropsychological Test Protocol for Sports-Related Return-to-Play Decision-Making. *Arch Clin Neuropsychol*, 2003. 18(3): 293–316.

Erlanger, D. M., et al., Neuropsychology of Sports-Related Head Injury: Dementia Pugilistica to Post Concussion Syndrome.*Clin Neuropsychol*, 1999. 13(2): 193–209.

Schatz, P., Long-Term Test-Retest Reliability of Baseline Cognitive Assessments Using ImPACT. *Am J Sports Med.* 38(1): 47–53.

Zohar, O., et al., Closed-Head Minimal Traumatic Brain Injury Produces Long-Term Cognitive Deficits in Mice. *Neuroscience*, 2003. 118(4): 949–55.

7

THE ACUTE ASSESSMENT AND MANAGEMENT OF SPORT-RELATED CONCUSSION: WHAT DO I DO WHEN AN ATHLETE SUSTAINS A CONCUSSION?

Mixed martial arts fighters B. J. Penn and Caol Uno were nearly identical in weight at 154 and 153 pounds respectively. Penn was approximately two inches taller. At the time, Uno had more experience. No one expected that the fight between them which was held on 2001 would last only 10 seconds.

In an exciting, energy filled start, Uno sprinted across the ring as soon as the bell rang. He leaped in the air and tried to connect a flying kick to Penn's face. But Penn brushed it aside, and advanced toward his opponent. Only seven seconds into the fight, Penn landed a left jab on the chin of Uno, twisting Uno's head rapidly to his left. Caol Uno stumbled backward, dazed, disoriented, off balance, stunned. He fell to the canvas where Penn unleashed a flurry of powerful rights to Uno's face until referee Larry Landless was forced to jump in and end the fight, a mere 10 seconds after it started.

Caol Uno was concussed.

Many readers will have seen similar knockouts during boxing or mixed martial arts bouts. But few will know what happens after the match. Few will know how a concussion should be responded to medically. Few will know what to do if a concussion occurs.

This chapter discusses an ideal approach to the assessment and management of sport-related concussions. It will review several different methods of evaluation and all the facets of care for an injured athlete. No program, physician or clinic will employ all of these resources, as many are simply different ways of doing the same thing. Only certain methods may be used by your caregivers, depending on the risk of concussion in a given sport, the available team resources, the knowledge and skill of personnel caring for athletes, and other factors. Often, sports medicine physicians, athletic trainers, internists, pediatricians, neuropsychologists, neurosurgeons, neurologists, and other medical personnel will use only some of these methods of evaluating athletes who have sustained concussions. For most concussions, which resolve readily without intervention, minimal therapy is all that will be required. Athletes who have more significant symptoms or longer recovery times may be referred to a specialty concussion clinic where a more complete evaluation may be performed and further therapies may be offered.

The assessment and management of concussion starts even before the first game of the season. Several measures, which can later be used to assess a potential injury, can be employed at the start of the season, before the athletes are at risk of sustaining a concussion.

It can be difficult for an athletic trainer or team physician to determine whether or not an athlete has sustained a concussion. Athletes often do not report their concussions to anyone. Some even lie about their symptoms when asked. In fact, a study of high school athletes conducted in 2004 by neuropsychologist Michael McCrea revealed that less than half of concussed athletes reported their injury. There are various reasons for this. Many do not recognize that their symptoms are due to a concussion. Even those who are knocked unconscious often do not recognize they have sustained a concussion. Many do not realize that a concussion is an injury to the brain. Since symptom reporting is a major part of diagnosing and managing a concussion, the lack of reporting makes it difficult for medical personnel to properly manage sport-related concussions. As noted, in order to help determine whether an athlete has sustained a concussion, athletic trainers or team physicians will often perform assessments of symptoms, balance, and brain function before the start of the season. These assessments can then be repeated in the event of a suspected concussion in order to assist these clinicians in making the diagnosis. They can be repeated further, to help monitor recovery.

Most sport-related concussion protocols will include the following assessments prior to the start of the season:

1. A symptom inventory
2. A balance assessment
3. A sideline concussion assessment tool
4. A neuropsychological assessment

Each of these is discussed further below.

SYMPTOM INVENTORIES

A symptom inventory is a measurement of the symptoms most often experienced by athletes after suffering a concussion. The most common symptom after a concussion is headache. Other common symptoms include insomnia, dizziness, amnesia, confusion, difficulty with memory, and difficulty concentrating. Figure 7.1 contains many of the symptoms associated with concussion. The symptom inventory will often be collected at the beginning of the season. It can be used in two ways. Some clinicians will ask athletes to report any symptoms they are having at the time of their baseline assessment. Thus, if they

Figure 7.1
An Example of a Symptom Inventory.

Post Concussion Symptom Scale

The following scale is to assess the symptoms which are due to your concussion. Please rate only those symptoms you have experienced in the last 24 hours.

	None	Mild		Moderate		Severe	
Headache	0	1	2	3	4	5	6
"Pressure in head"	0	1	2	3	4	5	6
Neck pain	0	1	2	3	4	5	6
Balance problems or dizziness	0	1	2	3	4	5	6
Nausea or vomiting	0	1	2	3	4	5	6
Vision problems	0	1	2	3	4	5	6
Hearing problems/ringing	0	1	2	3	4	5	6
"Don't feel right"	0	1	2	3	4	5	6
Feeling "dinged" or "dazed"	0	1	2	3	4	5	6
Confusion	0	1	2	3	4	5	6
Feeling slowed down	0	1	2	3	4	5	6
Feeling like "in a fog"	0	1	2	3	4	5	6
Drowsiness	0	1	2	3	4	5	6
Fatigue or low energy	0	1	2	3	4	5	6
More emotional than usual	0	1	2	3	4	5	6
Irritable	0	1	2	3	4	5	6
Difficulty concentrating	0	1	2	3	4	5	6
Difficulty remembering	0	1	2	3	4	5	6
Sadness	0	1	2	3	4	5	6
Nervous or anxious	0	1	2	3	4	5	6
Trouble falling asleep	0	1	2	3	4	5	6
Sleeping more than usual	0	1	2	3	4	5	6
Sensitivity to light	0	1	2	3	4	5	6
Sensitivity to noise	0	1	2	3	4	5	6
Other	0	1	2	3	4	5	6

had a headache, or were light-headed at the time of the baseline, they would record these symptoms. Other clinicians ask athletes to only record those symptoms that are due to a concussion. Thus, all athletes who were not recovering from a concussion at the time of their baseline assessment would rate a zero for all symptoms. Athletes asked to fill out a symptom inventory, should follow the instructions of the person administering it.

Although many symptom inventories exist, most are similar. Figure 7.1 is an example of the symptom inventory we use at the Sports Concussion Clinic in the Division of Sports Medicine at Children's Hospital Boston. It is based on the post-concussion symptom scale developed by the international conferences on concussion in sports.

BALANCE ASSESSMENT

There are several ways to perform balance assessments. Perhaps the easiest and most available method was described by the Third International Consensus on Concussion in Sports held in Zurich, November 2008. It is a modified version of the balance error scoring system developed by athletic trainer Kevin Guskiewicz and his colleagues. In order to perform the assessment, the examiner needs to have a stopwatch. Athletes are asked to perform three specific stances for 20 seconds each. Athletes should remove shoes, athletic taping, ankle braces, etc., prior to the start of the test.

The first stance requires athletes to stand with their hands on their hips, their feet together, and their eyes closed. The second stance requires athletes to stand on their nondominant foot. The dominant foot is the foot generally used to kick a ball. The opposite foot is known as the non-dominant foot. Since my preferred foot for kicking a ball is my right foot, my non-dominant foot would be my left one. Again, athletes must have their hands on their hips, their eyes closed, and must hold the stance steady for 20 seconds. The third and final stance requires athletes to stand with one foot in front of the other. In this position, the non-dominant foot is placed behind the dominant foot. Once again, athletes must place their hands on their hips, close their eyes and hold the stance for 20 seconds.

During each of three 20-second trials, an error is recorded for athletes if

1. Their hands are taken off of their hips.
2. They open their eyes.
3. They take a step, stumble, or fall.
4. They move their hip too far to one side.
5. They lift their toes or heel off of the ground.
6. They remain out of the stance for more than five seconds.

The total number of errors per trial is recorded, with the maximum allotted number of errors per stance being 10. The official balance examination score is 30 minus the number of errors recorded. For example, if an athlete has impeccable balance, and does not commit any errors, he would score a perfect 30. If another athlete opened her eyes during the first stance, stumbled during the second stance, lifted her heel off the ground later in the second stance, and performed perfectly in the third stance, she would have committed three total errors. Her final balance examination score would be 27.

There are other ways of assessing balance. Several machines can measure the amount of sway or rocking a person does when standing in certain positions. But these machines and the associated computer software can be fairly expensive. Often these are cost prohibitive for smaller, less well funded athletic programs. Even a television video game device known as the Wii Fit can be used to assess balance. In fact, the Wii Fit has even made its way into the medical literature in this regard. But currently, the modified Balance Error Scoring System is the most thoroughly studied, most easily understood, and most readily available for use in managing sport-related concussions. It is best used, by obtaining a baseline BESS score, prior to the start of the season, when an athlete is healthy. Then, repeated scores after a concussion can be used to monitor recovery.

Sideline Concussion Assessment Tools

It can often be unclear when a concussion has occurred. Athletes do not always recognize the signs and symptoms of concussion. Even when they know they have sustained a concussion, they are often reluctant to report it for fear of losing playing time, their position on the team, the respect of their teammates, the respect of their coach, their reputation for toughness, and various other reasons. Even when athletes report signs and symptoms such as headaches, light-headedness and poor balance during a game, it can be difficult sometimes to tell whether the athlete has sustained a concussion or the symptoms are due to something else, like dehydration. Sideline concussion assessment tools were developed in order to assist on-site medical personnel in diagnosing a sport-related concussion. They are intended to be used at the sideline or rink side during practice or competition when an athlete is suspected of having sustained a sport-related concussion. During practice and game times, athletes are often tired, sweaty, dehydrated, and distracted. Therefore, the best time to perform baseline sideline concussion assessments is in the middle or near the end of a practice. This helps account somewhat for these factors. There are several standardized sideline concussion assessment tools. We will discuss some of the more commonly used versions below.

Many readers will recall being struck in the head during athletics when they were younger. If you received any medical attention at all, it was likely a concerned parent, coach, or, if you were lucky, an athletic trainer. I remember this from when I was a kid. They might shine a light in your eyes. They might ask you your name, where you were, what day of the week it was, what time it was, or who the president was. These types of questions were designed to determine whether or not the athlete was "oriented" to person (who he or she was), place (where he or she was) and time (what day of the week and time of day it was). These were not difficult questions to answer, even for players who were concussed. Furthermore, the answers mattered little. Even when you got them wrong, people simply laughed and had you rest for a while, only to be returned to your sport later on that same day. At the time, concussion was not thought to be an injury of any consequence.

The Maddocks Questions

As we learned more about concussions, about the potential for complications after a concussion, about prolonged recoveries from concussions, and about the potential long-term effects of sustaining multiple concussions, sports medicine personnel started to develop better ways for determining whether or not an athlete had sustained a sport-related concussion. In 1995, an Australian named David Maddocks, out of the University of Melbourne, compared the answers to these questions, which assessed orientation, to the answers of questions regarding more immediate memory. His study was conducted on Australian rules football players who had sustained concussions. Specifically, the questions he used to judge recent memory were

1. At which ground (field) are we (playing)?
2. Which quarter is it?
3. How far into the quarter is it—first, middle, or last 10 minutes?
4. Which side kicked the last goal?
5. Which team did we play last week?
6. Did we win last week?

He found that concussed athletes found the questions pertaining to recent memory more difficult to answer than the questions used to determine general orientation. These questions have since come to be known as the "Maddocks" questions. They must be tailored for other sports. For example, to use them during an ice hockey match, one would have to replace "quarter" with "period." They are currently used by many sports medicine clinicians to help determine when an athlete has sustained a concussion.

They are included in the Sport Concussion Assessment Tool version 2 (SCAT 2) discussed further below.

Standardized Assessment of Concussion (SAC)

The Standardized Assessment of Concussion, or SAC, was developed by a neuropsychologist named Michael McCrea. This sideline assessment has four main components, used to assess orientation, immediate memory, concentration, and delayed recall (delayed memory). The general orientation component assesses whether or not the athlete is able to recall the month, date, day of the week, year, and approximate time of day. In the assessment of immediate memory, athletes are asked to recall a list of five words that were given to them by the examiner. While assessing concentration, athletes are asked to perform certain tasks, such as repeating a string of digits given to them by the examiner in reverse order. Reciting the months of the year in reverse order is another task for assessing concentration. In the delayed memory section, athletes are asked to recall the five words they were given previously. Each section is scored. The scores from each section are summed to give a total score. The test is meant to be performed at the start of the season. The preseason score serves as a baseline. Athletes suspected of having sustained a concussion repeat the test. Their post-injury score is then compared to their preseason baseline score.

Like all sideline assessment tools, the SAC is meant to be performed during a practice or competition in the event of a suspected concussion. Therefore, baseline scores should be obtained in similar circumstances, when an athlete has been working out and may be tired, may be mildly dehydrated, or may have decreased energy reserves, in order to simulate competition and practice conditions. Like the Maddocks questions, the SAC has also been incorporated into the Sport Concussion Assessment Tool version 2.

Sport Concussion Assessment Tool (SCAT and SCAT 2)

In 2004 a group of sport-related concussion experts met in Prague, Czech Republic, to "provide recommendations for the improvement of safety and health of athletes who suffer concussive brain injuries." In the summary and agreement statement from this meeting, the Sport Concussion Assessment Tool (SCAT) was published. It was developed by combining aspects of previous existing tools. The same group met again in Zurich, Switzerland in 2008, and updated the tool, publishing the second version, or Sport Concussion Assessment Tool 2 (SCAT 2), shown in Appendix 1. Designed to be used by medical and health professionals, the SCAT 2 contains the SAC and the Maddocks questions, discussed above., Because it is not subject to copyright restrictions, it is also available for free on the World Wide Web.

The SCAT 2 is the longest and most comprehensive of the sideline assessments. As noted, it incorporates several of the other available sideline assessments. It starts with a symptom inventory. It takes into account whether or not the athlete had gross imbalance or a loss of consciousness. It includes the Glasgow coma scale discussed in chapter 1, which is not useful in predicting recovery or long term effects from concussion but is highly useful in the immediate assessment of an acutely injured athlete. From there, it continues on to the Maddocks questions and Standardized Assessment of Concussion discussed above. It includes the modified Balance Error Scoring System and some well known neurological tests of physical coordination. The numbers of points athletes score on each section are added to yield a total, which can be compared to baseline scores. Finally, the SCAT 2 concludes with a summary and advice that can be given to the athlete. While these sideline assessment tools help medical personnel assess potential sport-related concussions, they are not used alone. A medical history, a physical examination, a symptom inventory, a sideline assessment, a balance assessment, and computerized neuropsychological testing should all be incorporated into a detailed concussion assessment and management protocol.

Often, sports medicine professionals will also ask athletes about their "concussion history" prior to the start of the season. A concussion history is a summary of any previous concussions, in or outside of sports, that the athlete has sustained. How many concussions the athlete has sustained, how long it took the athlete to recover from each, how each concussion occurred, when each concussion occurred, how significant the signs and symptoms of concussion were after each injury—these are all important details that will be used to determine management of future sport-related concussions. Many times, this concussion history will be obtained as part of the overall pre-participation physical examination.

Finally, a neuropsychological assessment should be performed on athletes prior to the start of the season. Although many sideline assessments include some neuropsychological tests as one of their components, these tests are brief and, at times, cursory. They consist of large or gross assessments of brain function. Many athletes, even after sustaining a sport-related concussion, will be able to perform the tasks required by these sideline assessments prior to being fully recovered. Therefore, more complete and thorough neuropsychological tests should be performed prior to the start of the season. Most often, these will be computerized neuropsychological assessments. Currently, there are several computerized neuropsychological assessments available for purchase. The most common ones are

- Immediate Post-concussion Assessment and Cognitive Testing (ImPACT)
- Concussion Resolution Index (CRI), developed by HeadMinder
- CogSport

Although much of the literature discussing computerized neuropsychological assessments includes the automated neuropsychological assessment metrics (ANAM), ANAM is used mainly by the U.S. Army Medical Department. At the time of this writing, I do not believe it is available for commercial use, although this may change in the future.

So, we now know some of the assessments and measurements that will be performed prior to the start of the season. These can be used to diagnose a concussion or monitor an athlete's recovery after a concussion. Let us now discuss what may happen when a concussion occurs.

Concussion is the most common brain injury in sports. But it is not the only one. Athletes can sustain skull fractures, often with bleeding in and around the brain. Even without a skull fracture athletes can suffer bleeding in and around the brain. They can suffer swelling of the brain. They can sustain a bruise of the brain. They can sustain a neck injury, including fractures of the cervical spine, which is the portion of the spine contained within the neck. Fractures of the cervical spine can be associated with damage to the spinal cord. Therefore, when an athlete sustains an injury to the head, the first concern of the medical team is not whether or not the athlete has a concussion. More immediate, time-sensitive issues need to be assessed for, evaluated, and treated, before consideration of a concussion. At the end of this chapter, I will present an example of an acute sports injury after a blow to the head, describing how it might be properly assessed and managed.

All personnel in the medical field are trained to respond to an acute injury in an organized fashion. The most pressing, emergent potential issues are assessed and treated immediately. Once all life-threatening issues have been addressed, the assessment continues, often focusing on less emergent injuries. An easy way clinicians use to remember the start of the emergency response is "A B C."

"A" stands for airway. When medical personnel arrive at the scene of an acutely injured athlete, the first task is to assess the airway. This means making sure that the mouth of the patient is open, and that nothing is blocking the flow of air from the mouth to the lungs. This is particularly important in an athlete who has sustained a head injury. When athletes are knocked unconscious, especially if they are lying on their backs, their tongue, tonsils, soft palate, other structures in the mouth, as well as objects such as tobacco products, chewing gum, teeth knocked loose at the time of impact, or mouth guards, may move to the back of the throat. These tissues and objects can block the flow of air from the mouth and nose to the lungs. This will prevent the patient from breathing. These tissues and objects must be cleared away from the airway, in order for the patient to breathe. As a result, you may see the athletic trainer, team physician, emergency medical technician or other medical response personnel remove the mouth guard, remove any other objects in the mouth, and position the patient's jaw in such a way that air can flow freely to the lungs.

For readers who have taken courses in first aid, wilderness medicine, or cardiopulmonary resuscitation (CPR), this may sound familiar. You may even recall some of the skills you were taught to reposition the airway. One of the more common is called the chin-lift maneuver. However, when an athlete is unconscious after an injury to the head, we do *not* perform the chin-lift maneuver. The chin-lift maneuver results in movement of the cervical spine. When athletes are unconscious after a blow to the head, they may have also injured or fractured their cervical spine. When the cervical spine is fractured, any inappropriate movement of the neck may make the fracture worse, and may result in damage to the spinal cord. Therefore, methods for clearing the airway that do not result in movement of the neck and cervical spine are preferred. Most commonly, the jaw-thrust technique is used.

In order to perform the jaw thrust maneuver, medical responders place their fingers behind the jaw bone, just underneath the ear lobes. The jaw is then pushed forward, such that the lower teeth move forward. The tongue and other tissues are brought forward with the jaw, thus clearing them from the airway, allowing air to pass through to the lungs, with minimal associated movement of the neck. Although this looks awkward and uncomfortable for the patient, it is a life-saving maneuver. It is important that parents, coaches, teammates and other caring spectators allow the medical team to do their work, without interfering. Any attempts to stop or interfere with the medical responders can result in catastrophic outcomes, including death and paralysis.

"B" is for breathing. Once the airway has been cleared of the tongue, other tissues, and other objects, the medical responder will make sure that the patient is breathing. Breathing is most often assessed by

1. Looking to see if the patient's chest is rising and falling as it typically does when a person breathes.
2. Listening for the sounds made in the chest when a person breathes. This may be accomplished by placing a stethoscope on the athlete's chest or by simply placing an ear directly against the athlete's chest.
3. Feeling for the rise and fall of the chest. This is most often accomplished by the medical responder resting his or her hand on the athlete's chest.
4. Feeling for the flow of air from the mouth. This can be accomplished by the medical responder placing his or her hand or cheek in front of the mouth and nose of the injured athlete.

If the athlete is not breathing, the medical responder will assist the patient with breathing. Again, there are several ways of doing this. One way is by giving rescue breaths or mouth-to-mouth resuscitation, where the medical responder seals his or her mouth with that of the athlete and blows air into the injured athlete's mouth, through the throat, and into the lungs. More commonly, the medical responder will place a mask over the mouth of the athlete. This mask is attached to a bag of air. When the bag is squeezed, air from inside the bag travels through the mask, into the patient's mouth, through the throat, and into the lungs.

Once the athlete is breathing, the medical responder will proceed to "C."

"C" is for circulation. Once it has been determined that an athlete's airway is clear and the athlete is breathing, the medical responder will assess for a heartbeat. This is most often accomplished by feeling for a pulse, either in the athlete's wrist or neck. If there is no pulse, the responder will try to pump blood from the heart to the rest of the body by performing "chest compressions." During chest compressions, the responder will apply pressure to the heart by pushing the portion of the athlete's chest that lies directly over the heart down several inches. This pressure is then released by letting go of the chest. When the heart is squeezed like this repeatedly, blood flows out of the heart, through the arteries, and supplies blood to the remainder of the body, including the brain. Again, it should be emphasized that while this appears awkward and uncomfortable for the athlete, it is a potentially life-saving technique.

Spectators must not interfere with emergency responders during one of these situations.

It should be noted that recent changes in these techniques have focused less on assisting breathing, and more on performing chest compressions to assist with circulation. The order of these responses may differ, depending on the current recommendations, the skills of the responder, the number of medical personnel available, and the immediate needs of the athlete.

Although the above assessment and resuscitation strategies can seem complex when reading about them, they can be performed quickly by trained and experienced personnel. In an athlete who is conscious, the airway, breathing, and circulation can be assessed simply by asking an athlete, "how are you?" If the athlete answers, then the medical responder knows that the airway is open, the athlete is breathing, and the heart is beating. Therefore, the remainder of the assessment can begin.

The remainder of the assessment after trauma is detailed and can seem complex to those unfamiliar with medical terminology and procedure. For the reader who is not medically trained, it would require an extensive discussion. Therefore, it is not included here. For those interested in learning more about the medical response to trauma, several articles and books are available and included in the suggested readings section at the end of this chapter.

A NOTE TO THE MEDICALLY TRAINED: For those readers who have taken courses in cardiopulmonary resuscitation or other medical interventions I would like to add a word of caution. Many athletic events will have medical personnel on the scene. These medical professionals will be well trained in the assessment and management of patients who sustain trauma. In addition, those who routinely cover these events will be well trained and knowledgeable about the unique injuries sustained by athletes and the unique techniques that must be used to assess and manage athletes. The response to trauma and resuscitation of athletes differs in several ways from the response to and resuscitation of other patients. In particular, athletes wearing bulky padding and athletic equipment, must be managed according to different protocols than non-athletes who sustain trauma. If such medical personnel are present, it is best to allow them to do their work without interfering. Many spectators who are medically trained will want to help or assist in these situations. Unless they have particular experience in the response to an injured athlete, however, they are more likely to cause harm than to be helpful. I have seen many well-meaning nurses and other medically trained spectators delay treatment and create unnecessary chaos during the response to an injured athlete by trying to assist.

Many times, an athlete who sustains a blow to the head shows more subtle signs or experiences more subtle symptoms, than those requiring the responses described above. If it is clear early in the evaluation that there are no signs or symptoms of bleeding in the brain, cervical spine injury, swelling of the brain, or other emergent issues, the medical responder then focuses on whether or

A NOTE ABOUT NECK AND CERVICAL SPINE INJURIES: As mentioned previously, the "cervical spine" refers to the bones of the spine that reside within the neck. Nerves cells originating in the brain travel through the neck, forming what is known as the spinal cord. The spinal cord descends from the brain through the neck and down the back. It sends nerves to the various parts of the body. Fractures and other injuries to the cervical spine can damage the spinal cord, resulting in serious, permanent neurological injury. Athletes who sustain fractures and other injuries to the cervical spine, can suffer permanent paralysis or even death. Therefore, the medical response team takes great care to avoid unnecessary movement of the neck while responding to and resuscitating an injured athlete. This concern is heightened in the athlete who sustained a sport related concussion associated with a change in mental status, confusion, or loss of consciousness.

not the athlete has sustained a concussion. Often, it is obvious that the player has sustained a concussion. But sometimes it is not. The medical team may use some of the preseason assessments discussed above to decide whether or not an athlete has sustained a concussion.

In a conscious athlete, medical personnel will often start by determining whether or not the athlete is oriented. As described previously, the term "orientation" refers to a person's understanding of his or her current surroundings and circumstances, often focusing on person, place, and time: Do athletes know 1) who they are, 2) where they are, and 3) what time of day, week, month, or year it is? In order to test an athlete's orientation, medical personnel often ask some basic questions such as

- What is your name?
- Where are you right now?
- What time of day is it?
- What day of the week is it?
- What is today's date?
- Who is the president of the United States?

This gives on-site medical personnel an immediate, but very broad, general insight into an injured athlete's brain functioning. The athlete's failure to answer these basic questions correctly can be a sign of serious injury, and will often prompt a more urgent medical response. If an athlete is oriented, the medical responder will often assess for the signs and symptoms of concussion. As a review, the signs and symptoms of concussion are listed in Tables 7.1 and 7.2. Remember, the word *symptoms* refers to the characteristics of illness that are felt or experienced by the patient. Things like headache, nausea, feeling "out of it," and sensitivity to light are all symptoms of a concussion. The word *signs* refers to the characteristics of illness which can be seen by those observing the patients. Unconsciousness, disorientation, confusion, and poor balance are all signs of a concussion.

Table 7.1
Common Signs of Concussion.

Signs of Concussion

• Loss of consciousness
• Amnesia, or forgetfulness
• Walking off-balance
• Acting disoriented
• Appearing dazed
• Acting confused
• Forgetting game rules or play assignments
• Inability to recall score or opponent
• Inappropriate emotionality
• Poor physical coordination
• Slow verbal responses
• Personality changes

By looking at these tables, one can see that many of the signs and symptoms of concussion are associated with other illnesses or medical conditions. Dehydration, which is common during athletic competition, can cause headaches, dizziness, and sensitivity to light. In order to help distinguish whether or not an athlete's signs and symptoms are due to concussion versus some other

Table 7.2
Common Symptoms of Concussion.

Symptoms of Concussion

• Headache
• Dizziness
• Difficulty concentrating
• Nausea or vomiting
• Difficulty balancing
• Vision changes
• Sensitivity to light
• Sensitivity to noise
• Feeling "out of it"
• Ringing in the ears
• Drowsiness
• Sadness

medical condition, medical personnel will often focus on the facts surrounding the onset of symptoms. For example, if an athlete skates off of the ice during a hockey game and tells the athletic trainer he feels light-headed and has a headache, the athletic trainer will often ask the athlete a series of questions:

1. When did the headache start?
2. Did it come on gradually or did it start suddenly?
3. Were you struck in the head at the time the headache started?
4. Do you feel nauseous?
5. Have you ever felt this way before?
6. How did you feel before the game started?

The answers to these initial questions will often lead to other questions. The object is to get a full understanding of how the symptoms started, and how they have the changed since they started. For example, the athlete may report that he awoke late for class that day and skipped breakfast. He had a chicken sandwich for lunch without a drink. He was mildly light-headed when he stood up initially for his line change during the first period. He noticed a small headache during the intermission between first and second period. It has since progressed. He has not sustained any major body checks or blows to the head.

In this case, the athletic trainer may conclude the athlete is likely dehydrated. He may be offered a sports drink or even intravenous fluids. He may be allowed to continue playing.

Alternatively, the athlete may report that he felt well all game until he sustained an open-ice body check that lifted him off of his feet, causing him to land head first on the ice. He experienced the immediate onset of headaches. He rose up to finish the play and noticed he was light-headed for the first time that day. He skated off the ice and reported to the athletic trainer.

In this case, the athletic trainer might conclude that the athlete has sustained a concussion. He would be removed from play and further assessment would begin.

Typically, medical personnel will assess for signs and symptoms of other potential injuries discussed above, such as bleeding in or around the brain, swelling of the brain, and neck or cervical spine injury. If there were no other injuries, then medical personnel might use one of the symptoms inventories or sideline assessments discussed above to help decide whether or not an athlete has sustained a concussion. Sometimes, this will be unnecessary, as the diagnosis can be made without the use of these preseason evaluations.

Once the diagnosis of concussion has been made, the athlete should be removed from play immediately. Continuing to play with a concussion places the athlete at risk for a prolonged recovery, more pronounced deficits in brain functioning, and catastrophic injuries such as second impact syndrome.

Once concussed athletes have been removed from play, they should be monitored for the next few hours. As was mentioned earlier, concussion is the most common neurological injury in sports. But it is not the only one. Swelling of the brain, bleeding into or around the brain, and bruising of the brain may not always be apparent immediately after injury. Occasionally, more extensive damage to the brain will not be detectable or obvious until minutes to hours later. Therefore, athletes who have sustained a suspected sport-related concussion should be observed closely and monitored, with designated personnel checking on them every 15 to 20 minutes for the first few hours after injury. Often, these neurological checks will be performed by the athletic trainer or team physician while the athlete remains at field side, rink side, or at the arena. However, when the contest is over and all athletes are leaving the area of play, others may be asked to perform monitoring and observation of the athlete. Teammates, roommates, family members, and others should be asked to monitor the patient over the first 24 hours. Any concerning signs or symptoms should prompt the athlete to seek emergency medical attention.

Some of the signs and symptoms of more extensive brain injury are

- persistent vomiting or the new onset of vomiting
- somnolence, where the athlete appears sleepy and is difficult to rouse
- persistent confusion, disorientation, or the new onset of confusion or disorientation
- seizure
- appearing abnormal

Although "appearing abnormal" is a vague phrase, it is meant to be so. It can be difficult to describe exactly what it is abnormal about a traumatically brain injured athlete. But most people can tell when something is wrong. Most people have an intuitive sense, an innate ability, to determine sick from nonsick, worrisome from not worrisome. If ever you get the sense that something is concerning about an athlete suspected of having sustained a sport-related concussion, seek immediate medical attention. It is better to raise the alarm, if only to find out that the athlete has a concussion from which he or she will recover completely than to miss a potentially catastrophic brain injury.

Athletes will recover from concussions spontaneously. At present, there is no medication or other therapy that is proven to treat concussion. However, there are some steps athletes can take to avoid worsening of their symptoms and, perhaps, to help them recover faster.

Physical Rest

After athletes sustain a concussion, they are immediately removed from sports. Many people believe this is solely so that they won't hit their heads again and sustain another concussion. However, there is another reason for removing the athlete from sport. For many athletes, physical exertion makes their symptoms worse. Even noncontact activities such as running, ice skating, weight lifting, and working out on exercise machines will often make symptoms worse and, perhaps, prolong recovery. That means that it may take longer for athletes to recover from their concussions if they are exercising. So as soon as an athlete has been diagnosed with a concussion, he or she should be removed from all forms of training and exercise. This will treat the symptoms and, perhaps, help athletes to recover faster.

COGNITIVE REST

The Merriam-Webster dictionary defines cognitive as "of, relating to, being, or involving conscious intellectual activity (as thinking, reasoning, or remembering)." Cognitive processes are those that involve thinking, remembering, concentrating, or reasoning. Cognitive rest requires avoiding cognitive activities such as reading, writing, doing homework, playing games such as chess or Trivial Pursuit, playing video games, text messaging, working online, and so forth. Often the symptoms of an athlete recovering from a concussion will get worse during these activities. Engaging in cognitive activities may delay recovery from a concussion. Athletes should be encouraged to avoid cognitive activities while they are recuperating from a sport-related concussion.

For student athletes, this can be quite difficult. When in school, an athlete is required to perform cognitive activities on a daily basis. Nearly all schoolwork requires reading, writing, reasoning, remembering and concentrating. Therefore, I often recommend athletes stay home from school for several days immediately following a sport-related concussion. While missing school is never ideal, students will miss school on various occasions, such as when they have the flu, when they are vomiting, when a parent takes them on a vacation, and for many other reasons. Certainly, missing several days of school in order to recover from a traumatic brain injury is warranted. I recommend no more than five days of absence from school. Many athletes will be fully or nearly symptom-free at that point. In fact, nearly 85 percent of high school athletes report being completely symptom-free and are deemed by their athletic trainer to be recovered within a week after their injury. The time until recovery is even shorter for older athletes. Concussed athletes will note significant improvement in their symptoms after the first several days if they truly rest themselves, avoiding both physical and cognitive exertion. Therefore, no other treatments will be necessary to treat the majority of sport-related concussions.

Steps to take if you suspect an athlete has sustained a sport-related concussion:

1. Remove the athlete from play immediately.
2. Take the athlete directly to on-site medical personnel so they can evaluate the athlete, check for other potential injuries, administer any needed treatments, and instruct you further.

3. If there is no on-site medical personnel, take the athlete to a doctor, or, if necessary, call for an ambulance.
4. If medical personnel diagnose the athlete with a concussion, check on the athlete every 15–20 minutes for the first few hours after injury. If you see anything concerning, call a doctor or, if necessary, an ambulance.
5. Encourage physical and cognitive rest as described above. This should start immediately and should include an absence from school for the first few days if the athlete is not feeling better.
6. Schedule an appointment with the athlete's primary care physician, or, if the athlete has already been diagnosed with a concussion as opposed to another illness or injury, a clinician with experience in the assessment and management of sport-related concussions.

In order to help illustrate some of the points made above, an example of how an acutely injured athlete might be evaluated and managed on site is provided here.

Kevin is a 15-year-old football player for a local high school. Although only a sophomore, he is both fast and strong for his age. He often plays with the varsity football team. It is late in the third quarter. Kevin's team is winning by three points. He has been playing on both sides of the ball, participating in both offense and defense. Currently, his team is on offense. They have driven down the field to his opponents' 17-yard line. As Kevin is the strongest running back on the team, the coach puts him in. It's third down. They need a total of four yards to get another first down. The ball is snapped. The quarterback turns to his left and fakes a handoff to the halfback. He then pitches back to Kevin. Kevin takes the ball, lowers his shoulder, and follows the halfback toward the defensive line. The halfback attempts to block one of the oncoming defenseman. However, he is run down and Kevin is struck simultaneously by two on-rushing defenders. Kevin's helmet collides with that of one of his opponents. He is knocked backward to the ground. The back of his head bounces off the turf.

Kevin's teammates immediately realize something is wrong. He is not moving on the ground. He makes no effort to stand up. They rush to his side and frantically wave for the coach and athletic trainer to come on to the field. When the athletic trainer arrives, he sees that Kevin is lying on the ground motionless, not responding to his name. The athletic trainer sends two of the other players and one of the assistant coaches to call for an ambulance.

Immediately the athletic trainer takes what looks like a pair of pliers from his bag. He cuts the two rubber bands on the side of Kevin's helmet which hold the face mask in place. He removes the face mask from the helmet and puts it aside. He removes Kevin's mouth guard, and opens his mouth. Seeing that there are no other objects in Kevin's mouth, he listens to see whether or not Kevin is breathing. However he is unable to hear Kevin's breath sounds through his jersey, shoulder pads, and breastplate. He quickly removes a pair of scissors from his medical bag. He cuts Kevin's jersey straight down the middle and down each of the sleeves. He cuts the laces at the center of Kevin's breastplate as well as the straps around his arms. He opens the breastplate, exposing Kevin's chest. He places his ear on the chest and is able to hear Kevin breathing both on the right and left sides of his chest. He sees that Kevin's chest rises on both the left and right sides. He then holds Kevin by the wrist, feeling for a pulse, which he notes is present and strong. He moves to Kevin's head, grasps his helmet on either side, and prevents any movement of Kevin's head and neck.

Two additional athletic trainers arrive around the same time as the ambulance. The emergency medical technicians place a large plastic board at Kevin's side. The emergency medical technicians and an athletic trainer each line up on Kevin's right side. When the athletic trainer who is holding Kevin's head counts to three, they roll Kevin up on his side. One of the other athletic trainers slides the plastic board up against Kevin's side, in the space where he was just lying. Again, the athletic trainer holding Kevin's head counts to three. They roll him onto his back, such that he is now lying on top of the hard plastic board. They attempt to place a hard plastic collar around Kevin's neck. Realizing that they cannot place the collar safely, because Kevin's helmet and shoulder pads are in the way, they place the collar aside on the ground. Using the previously cut laces of Kevin's breastplate, as well as some athletic tape, they re-secure his shoulder pads to his body. Two padded blocks are placed on either side of Kevin's neck. His helmet, shoulder pads, and the remainder of his body are secured to the hard, plastic board using webbing straps. The board is lifted and placed into the ambulance. Kevin is transported to a local emergency department.

On the way to the hospital, Kevin wakes up. He is clearly anxious and somewhat confused. He does not understand why he is in an ambulance. He is visibly anxious. He continues to ask the ambulance driver where his parents are. He is told multiple times what occurred at the field and that he is on his way to an emergency department. He continues to ask where his parents are. When he arrives in the emergency department Kevin is much calmer. He is still somewhat confused. He is able to tell doctors that he was playing in a football game earlier that day. He does not, however, recall the injury. He does realize he is in an emergency department but cannot recall which city he is in. Ultimately, his football helmet and shoulder pads are removed very carefully by the nurses and doctors in the emergency department, such that they do not cause significant movement of his head or neck. He is placed in a hard plastic collar.

The doctor in the emergency department asks Kevin multiple questions. He spends several minutes examining Kevin and having him perform various tasks. During the examination Kevin's parents arrive. The doctor explains to them that Kevin was injured during today's football game. Although he is somewhat disoriented, he otherwise appears well. The doctor tells his parents that as a precaution he will be observed in the emergency department to ensure that he does not have any signs or symptoms of other injuries to the brain or neck. If he develops any concerning signs or symptoms, the doctor explains, they will likely get a picture of Kevin's brain known as a "head CT."

Kevin is admitted to the hospital. Periodically throughout the night nurses and doctors come in and wake Kevin, ask him some questions, and examine him. Over *the course of the evening and the following morning he returns back to normal. He is able to answer all questions. He is able to perform all the tasks asked by the doctors examining him. The doctors feel the back of Kevin's neck and ask if he has any pain or tenderness there. He does not. They loosen the collar from around his neck and ask him to slowly move his head in all different directions, instructing him to stop if he develops any pain or unusual sensations. Kevin is able to look all around the room without any difficulty, pain, tenderness, or other unusual sensations. The plastic collar is removed. Although Kevin continues to complain of headaches and difficulty concentrating, he and his parents are informed that this is typical after a concussion. They expect that these symptoms will resolve over the next several days to weeks. They discharge him to home, instructing him to follow up with a specialist in sport-related concussion over the next week or two. They instruct him to avoid all physical activity, exercising, and football until he sees the specialist. The doctors also recommend he avoids school, homework, reading, playing video games, working online, and any other forms of cognitive activity.*

Several things are worth noting about the above example:

1. Once the athletic trainer had access to Kevin and confirmed that 1) his airway was open, 2) he was breathing, and 3) he had a pulse, he immediately focused his attention on ensuring that Kevin's head and neck did not move more than necessary. As discussed above, injuries to the cervical spine and spinal cord can be devastating. Therefore, this is one of the top priorities of medical personnel responding to an injured athlete once it has been established that the airway is open, the athlete is breathing, and that the athlete has a pulse.

2. When Kevin is placed on the hard plastic board for transport to the emergency department, it is the athletic trainer holding his head and neck in place who controls his movements by directing the rest of the team when and how to move Kevin, and by counting to three in order to coordinate the timing of each movement. This is standard medical practice. Since it is of utmost importance to minimize any inappropriate movements of the injured athlete's head and neck, the person controlling the head and neck determines when all movements take place. Typically, the medical provider will instruct the other medical personnel to move the patient in a specific way "on the count of three."

3. Kevin was placed in the ambulance and transported to the emergency department without a hard collar placed on his neck. While this may seem surprising to readers with some medical training, this is the ideal way to transport an athlete with helmets and shoulder pads that inhibit the placement of a hard neck collar. Multiple medical studies have shown that attempting to place a hard neck collar, also known as a cervical collar, on an athlete wearing helmets and shoulder pads can result in significant movement and poor alignment of the bones of the neck. This movement increases the athlete's risk for catastrophic outcome such as spinal cord injury. Although there are situations in which the helmets and shoulder pads need to be removed on site, they are rare. When the shoulder pads and helmet need to be removed, then a hard neck collar should be placed. In ideal circumstances, the athlete will be transported wearing both the helmet and the shoulder pads.

4. Kevin did not receive a computed tomogram of the head, more commonly known as a head CT. Many parents, other concerned relatives, and friends of the athlete will want to be absolutely sure that there is no bleeding or swelling of the brain. Many more will be under the impression that a doctor can "see" a concussion on a head CT. Therefore, they will often ask for a head CT. Certainly, many athletes who present to an emergency department after sustaining an injury to the head will require a head CT in order to make sure that there are no such injuries to the brain. However, in order to obtain the pictures of the brain that make up the head CT, the brain is exposed to radiation. Therefore, a great deal of thought is put into deciding whether or not an injured athlete requires a head CT. The amount of radiation to which the athlete is exposed during a head CT is a relatively small. Therefore, if the emergency medicine physician treating you or your athlete feels a head CT is warranted, you should not worry about this small amount of radiation. However, if the doctor in the emergency department does not believe a head CT is indicated, then it is better not to have one. The decision to obtain or not obtain a head CT is best left to the doctors examining the injured athlete.

5. When Kevin is discharged from the hospital the doctors who cared for him during his hospital stay instructed him to avoid physical exertion, cognitive exertion, and football, until he is cleared to resume these activities by a physician with expertise in assessing and managing sport-related concussions. This is an ideal situation. However, with the enormous amount of medical literature produced every day, and the speed with which medical recommendations change in response to new discoveries, it is impossible for all physicians to be up to date and well informed regarding all illnesses and injuries. Therefore, the doctor caring for your athlete may make recommendations based on older medical guidelines. This should not alarm you. This is not reflective of the physician's intelligence or medical capabilities. It simply reflects the rapid speed of medical science and the enormous volumes of information in the medical literature. Doctors need to prioritize those medical issues that are of greatest importance for their practice. For physicians working in the emergency department or in the hospital, it is most important to make sure that any emergent issues are realized and treated. Therefore, this will be the focus of their efforts. This will be the medical literature with which they will be most familiar. After leaving the hospital, you should schedule a follow-up appointment with your primary care physician, a sports medicine physician, or other clinician experienced in the assessment and management of sport-related concussions. These doctors can give you the up-to-date information on recovering from a sport-related concussion.

In summary, the assessment of sport-related concussions should start prior to the start of the season by obtaining baseline measurements of athletes' symptoms, balance, and neurocognitive function. There are several available tools to help clinicians make and record these measurements. When a suspected concussion occurs, the first priority of the responding medical providers is to make sure there are no emergent injuries that require immediate assessment and management. Once any emergent issues have been addressed, medical providers will determine whether or not a concussion has occurred. Athletes who have sustained a sport-related concussion should be immediately put on both physical and cognitive rest. They should be monitored for the first 24 hours after injury, and monitored closely by a clinician for the first few hours after injury. Any concerning signs or symptoms should result in immediate medical attention. Most athletes will recover from sport-related concussion quickly, within days to weeks, requiring only physical and cognitive rest in order to fully recover.

SUGGESTED READINGS

American College of Sugeons. *Advanced Trauma Life Support for Doctors, Student Manual, 8th Edition.*

Banerjee, R., M. A. Palumbo, and P. D. Fadale, Catastrophic Cervical Spine Injuries in the Collision Sport Athlete, Part 2: Principles of Emergency Care. *Am J Sports Med*, 2004. 32(7): 1760–64.

Concussion (Mild Traumatic Brain Injury) and the Team Physician: A Consensus Statement. *Med Sci Sports Exerc*, 2006. 38(2): 395–99.

Guskiewicz, K. M., S. E. Ross, and S. W. Marshall, Postural Stability and Neuropsychological Deficits after Concussion in Collegiate Athletes. *J Athl Train*, 2001. 36(3): 263–73.

Harris, M. B. and R. K. Sethi, The Initial Assessment and Management of the Multiple-Trauma Patient with an Associated Spine Injury. *Spine* (Phila Pa 1976), 2006. 31(Suppl 11): S9–15; discussion S36.

McCrea, M., et al., Standardized Assessment of Concussion in Football Players. *Neurology*, 1997. 48(3): 586–88.

McCrea, M., et al., Unreported Concussion in High School Football Players: Implications for Prevention. *Clin J Sport Med*, 2004. 14(1): 13–17.

Swartz, E. E., et al., National Athletic Trainers' Association Position Statement: Acute Management of the Cervical Spine-Injured Athlete. *J Athl Train*, 2009. 44(3): 306–31.

8

POTENTIAL THERAPIES: WHAT CAN BE DONE TO HELP MY ATHLETE RECOVER?

On May 26, 2010, the Boston Celtics were playing the Orlando Magic in Game 5 of the Eastern Conference finals. Orlando center Dwight Howard pulled up for a shot. As he descended, his left elbow struck the Celtics forward Glen "Big Baby" Davis in the face. Davis lay on the ground for several seconds, staring into space. His first attempt to stand resulted in his simply lifting his head and shoulders up, only to relax back shortly. The second time he attempted to stand, he scurried along on all fours, unable to get his feet underneath his large, powerful frame. When he was finally able to get to his feet, he stumbled off to his left, visibly off balance, away from the play, until he collapsed into the arms of an official. His teammates came to support him. But he was so unsteady on his feet, he ultimately was placed on the ground to be assessed by the team's sports medicine staff.

Glen Davis was concussed.

As with most concussed athletes, Glen Davis was prescribed physical rest, which not only kept him from sustaining another injury to the head but also hastened his recovery.

While most athletes will recover quickly from their sport-related concussions, some will have a more prolonged recovery period. Approximately 2 percent of high school athletes who sustain a sport-related concussion will have symptoms that last longer than a month. Some of these athletes will take many months to recover, even up to a year. For this unfortunate minority, there are many other considerations.

PHYSICAL REST

As noted previously, physical rest is one of the ways concussed athletes can help themselves feel better and recovery more quickly. Avoiding physical activity for the first several days is usually not much of an issue or challenge. More prolonged periods away from exercise, however, can be challenging.

Athletes who are in school must be excused from gym class. This will often require a note from a physician. If possible, recess should be allowed, but monitored, so that the athlete is safe, without an increased risk of trauma to the head or over-exertion leading to an exacerbation of symptoms. Under no circumstances should athletes be cleared for return to contact or collision sports before they are completely recovered from their concussions.

In addition to the avoidance of exercise, increasing the amount of time spent sleeping may help athletes who sustain a sport-related concussion recover faster. If an athlete typically sleeps 8 hours per night, increasing to 10 or more hours a night may help with recovery. Some athletes find sleeping for such a long period difficult. In those cases, taking a nap during the day may help the athlete get some extra sleep during his or her recovery. Unfortunately, insomnia, which is an inability to obtain adequate sleep, is a common symptom of concussion. Thus, while increased amounts of sleep may assist with recovery, they can be hard to obtain. Some strategies for addressing insomnia are discussed below.

Most athletes enjoy exercise. It improves their mood, their health, their self-image. In such athletes, a prolonged absence from physical activity can lead to depression and irritability. When this occurs, counseling with a sports psychologist is often effective. Through counseling, these symptoms can be alleviated; and athletes can learn coping strategies to help them deal with their injuries. Occasionally, medications can be considered.

If the recovery period is markedly prolonged, lasting several months, physicians will occasionally allow some athletes to engage in mild aerobic activity as long as 1) it does not increase the athlete's risk for injury to the head and 2) it does not make the athlete's symptoms worse. This is a completely reasonable practice. Not all concussions are the same. Similarly, the recovery from concussion is not always the same. Athletes who have been recovering from a concussion for greater than a month and wish to engage in some exercise should discuss this possibility with the clinician managing their concussion.

COGNITIVE REST

As discussed in the previous chapter, cognitive activities, those that require thinking, remembering, concentrating, or reasoning, should be avoided during recovery from a concussion. This will often necessitate an absence from school. Usually, this can be accomplished without too much trouble for the first few days after injury. Some athletes, however, will have symptoms that last longer than the first week after their injury. For these athletes, I recommend they return to school, but with some assistance and with academic accommodations. Academic accommodations are discussed further below.

But first, many people ask, why not keep athletes out of school until they are completely recovered? There are several reasons why I advise against this practice. Athletes learn more in school than simply the subjects in which they are enrolled. They learn to make friends, respect authority, manage a schedule, interact with their peers, and socialize. Much of this is learned through less formal means than classroom teaching itself, and can be learned without excessive cognitive exertion. Furthermore, although many young athletes do not readily admit it, school is fun. This is where they see their friends and where most of their social interactions take place. Learning social skills is essential. In fact, I would argue that learning social skills is ultimately more important in life than learning the classroom subjects. Don't get me wrong, learning mathematics, reading, writing, English grammar, science, and other core subjects is extremely important. But you can be the most knowledgeable person in the world, and if you have poor social skills, no one will want to work with you. You will find it hard to get a job, and even harder to be successful at one. Those who learn to treat others with respect, to interact with teammates and classmates, to respect authority, and to stand up for themselves while still being agreeable, are more pleasant to work with. Thus, they often have an easier time finding a job, and being successful at a given job.

Reentering into school while still recovering from a concussion, however, is not an easy task. Schoolwork and homework require the very same activities that make symptoms worse: remembering, reasoning, concentrating, and thinking. Furthermore, the concussed brain is not functioning properly. The speed with which a concussed athlete is able to process information is reduced. The ability to concentrate is decreased. Reaction time is slowed. Memory is poor. Therefore, concussed athletes often have difficulties in school and their grades suffer accordingly.

In order to help them stay in school, keep up with their course work, and minimize any negative impacts their concussion might otherwise have on their grades, concussed athletes are entitled to academic accommodations. These should be put in place as soon as it becomes clear the athlete will not recover quickly. Academic accommodations are exceptions to the normal school rules and timetables that allow concussed athletes to reenter school prior to complete recovery. Some of the more commonly used accommodations are

1. Giving concussed students preprinted class notes, so they can listen to the teacher during class, as opposed to concentrating on both listening to the teacher and copying down all of the information for later reference.
2. Giving concussed athletes extra time on tests and quizzes. Since the speed with which concussed athletes are able to process information has been slowed, and the memory of concussed athletes is temporarily diminished, it takes longer to complete tasks that they were able to complete rather quickly prior to the injury. Thus, extra time is required to take tests and quizzes during recovery.
3. Offering concussed athletes tutors to help them with their homework. Many students who have not sustained a concussion take advantage of tutoring. During recovery from a concussion, tutoring may be helpful.
4. Allowing the athlete to go to the nurse's office to lie down if concussion symptoms increase during the school day. Even with academic accommodations in place, school attendance can exacerbate symptoms. Rest will help relieve them.

5. Reducing the athlete's work load.
6. Offering concussed athletes extensions on their homework assignments. As discussed, athletes recovering from a concussion will often need more time to accomplish tasks that once came to them quite readily. Similarly, they will need to take breaks when their symptoms increase. This prolongs the time needed to complete assignments. Thus, extensions on these assignments allow the athletes to complete them properly, and to the best of their capabilities.
7. Some athletes will need to limit their course load. Rather than taking six or seven courses at a time, some athletes might only be able to manage two to four courses at a time. They might only attend a half day of school as opposed to a whole day. When this is necessary, I recommend athletes maintain courses that build upon themselves, such as mathematics and science. You cannot learn how to multiply two numbers each containing multiple digits, unless you have first learned to multiply two single integers together. Mathematics generally builds on itself in this way. It can be difficult to return to math class in March if you missed the material covered in February. Classes like English and history tend to be somewhat more forgiving. You can read *Animal Farm*, even if you have never read *Oliver Twist*. Each novel can be read independently of the other.

There are several other strategies which may help athletes accomplish their schoolwork while recovering from a sport-related concussion. Many healthy, uninjured students will complete their homework for the day in one session. They will sit down at a desk or table for several hours straight and complete all of their assignments. While this is a perfectly reasonable way of doing it when healthy, such a long period of concentration, thinking, and reasoning will often exacerbate a concussed athlete's symptoms. A better approach during recovery is to accomplish homework assignments in small chunks of time. Doing one's homework in 20-minute intervals with 10–15 minute breaks in between may help prevent symptoms from worsening.

A few things should be remembered about academic accommodations. First, they are temporary. When an athlete has recovered, there is no longer a need for academic accommodations. They should then be discontinued. Second, academic accommodations are a two-edged sword. While they may seem advantageous to some readers, most athletes dislike them. The athlete is still responsible for the work covered in class. Academic accommodations allow for the forgiveness of some minor assignments, and allow the athlete to postpone more important assignments. But tests, quizzes, and major assignments need to be made up. And no athletes like the thought of making up weeks' worth of quizzes, tests, and homework assignments once they have recovered from their concussion.

Ultimately, the goal of academic accommodations is to allow concussed students to stay in school and keep up with their schoolwork as best as they can without 1) making their symptoms worse, 2) delaying their recovery more than necessary, and 3) allowing their grades to decline unnecessarily.

OTHER POTENTIAL THERAPIES

If you or your athlete is taking a long time to recover from a concussion despite full physical rest and full cognitive rest, consider seeing a specialist in the assessment and management of sport-related concussion. Although there is no medicine that has been shown to effectively speed the recovery form a concussive brain injury, many of the symptoms can be treated medically. Most physicians will be unfamiliar with these treatments. Many are still being developed, and therefore will be unknown to many clinicians. Seeing someone who specializes in the assessment and management of concussion may open up other possibilities for treatment. Some specific symptoms are discussed below.

Headache

Headache is the most common symptom of concussion in general and of sport-related concussion specifically. Often, headaches will resolve within the first few days to weeks after a sport-related concussion with only physical and cognitive rest, as discussed. But for some athletes, headaches will persist. Ironically, those who seem, at first, to have sustained only a minor injury, often suffer worse headaches afterward, and suffer headaches for a longer period of time, than those who initially seemed to have a more severe injury.

Obtaining physical and cognitive rest will help alleviate headaches caused by concussion. Avoiding prolonged periods of concentration, thinking, and reasoning can help prevent headaches. Therefore, much like the recommendations provided here for athletes in school, all athletes should try to break up cognitive tasks that they cannot avoid into many small chunks of time, as opposed to focusing on a given cognitive task for one long stretch of time.

In response to post-concussive headaches, many athletes will start taking common over-the-counter medications such as acetaminophen, ibuprofen, and aspirin. Certainly, these medications are useful for treating headaches in general. They are safe and well tolerated by most patients. However, they should not be taken routinely to treat the headaches of a sport-related concussion. They tend to be ineffective in treating post-concussive headaches. Oftentimes, athletes take these medications three or four times per day in an attempt to alleviate the headaches. Once an athlete has been taking these medications multiple times per day for several days or weeks, it can be hard to stop them. Any attempt to stop the medications will result in "rebound headaches." Rebound headaches are similar to withdrawal headaches. Many readers who enjoy coffee, tea, and other caffeinated beverages will be familiar with withdrawal headaches. Those who enjoy these drinks daily will often experience withdrawal headaches when they go a day without caffeine. Similarly, when concussed athletes taking acetaminophen, ibuprofen, or aspirin regularly for headaches try to stop the medications, they will experience a rebound headache. Athletes will often mistake these rebound headaches for persistent post-concussive headaches. This makes it difficult to determine when the athlete has recovered. Therefore, for the first few days to weeks after injury, I recommend athletes respond to the headaches by trying to obtain more rest, and by limiting their activities. Other medications are more effective for treating post-concussive headaches that do not resolve over the first few days to weeks, and therefore become a significant, daily problem.

If headaches persist, and are negatively impacting an athlete's quality of life, there are multiple other strategies and medications that can be used to treat the headaches related to a concussion. Oftentimes, at the Sports Concussion Clinic at Children's Hospital Boston, we will offer the athlete a medicine called amitriptyline. Amitriptyline is most commonly used as an antidepressant, or a medication given to patients who suffer from clinical depression. However, it is also effective at treating headaches: migraine headaches, tension headaches, cluster headaches, and post-concussive headaches. It has been studied specifically in patients who have headaches after sustaining a concussion. It decreases the frequency with which patients recovering from a concussion suffer headaches. It reduces the intensity of headaches, when they do occur, in patients recovering from a concussion. In fact, amitriptyline is so useful in treating post-concussive headaches that often a dose as small as one-tenth of the dose used to treat depression is effective in reducing the intensity and frequency of post-concussive headaches. At such a small dosages, amitriptyline tends to be well tolerated by patients. Side effects tend to be minimal. However, sleepiness is one side effect that is common, even at the small dosages used to treat post-concussive headaches. As many patients suffering from post-concussive headaches also have insomnia, this side effect can be advantageous. Amitriptyline can be used to treat both the headaches and the insomnia.

Although we commonly use the amitriptyline to treat post-concussive headaches, especially in younger athletes, there are many other potential therapies and medications that can be used to treat these headaches. Therapies such as biofeedback, psychotherapy, physical therapy, and trigger point injections can be used to treat post-concussive headaches, either by themselves or in conjunction with medications. Other medications that physicians may consider for the treatment of post-concussive headaches include beta-blockers, calcium channel blockers, valproic acid, triptans, topiramate, gabapentin, pregabalin, and dihydroergotamine. If you or your athlete has persistent headaches that negatively impact the quality of life for weeks after sustaining a sport-related concussion, you should discuss the best potential therapies for treating those headaches with the physician managing your sport-related concussion. Many times, prior to starting such medications, physicians will order further tests to assess for other potential injuries as well as the general health of the patient. This should not alarm you. Although it is not always necessary, these tests are commonly performed prior to starting new medications.

If the first one or two medications recommended fails to significantly alleviate the athlete's headaches, consultation with a headache specialist can sometimes be useful. Headache specialists are most often are neurologists. At the Sports Concussion Clinic at Children's Hospital Boston, we work closely with several neurologists who have significant experience and expertise in treating headaches. I often refer athletes to these neurologists if I am unable to control their headaches with the first one or two medications tried.

Insomnia

Insomnia is the ability to obtain adequate sleep. As it is common, many readers will have heard of insomnia or even experienced insomnia at some point in their lives. Insomnia is one of the most common symptoms of concussion, especially in athletes who do not recover quickly. There are several strategies for helping an athlete who is suffering from insomnia after a concussion to get some sleep.

The first and easiest strategy is to rid the athlete's bedroom of all potentially distracting items. Today's athletes are surrounded by distractions. Their bedrooms are often filled with electronics such as stereos, videogames, televisions, cell phones, laptop computers, iPods, and more. They are constantly bombarded with social messages through phone calls, text messages, instant messages, e-mails, Facebook messages, Myspace messages, etc. Eliminating such distractions from the bedroom and having the athlete lie down in a quiet, dark room will help induce sleep. Simply turning these gadgets off or switching them to vibrate is less effective. The mere presence of these devices can be distracting. Not only electronics should be removed. The presence of a to-do list, schedule, or daily planner can bring to mind all the tasks that lay ahead. This can cause stress and anxiety, which prevents sleep.

Similarly, concussed athletes suffering from insomnia should avoid potential stimulants such as caffeine or nicotine. Alcohol may also cause difficulties sleeping. For this, as well as other reasons, an athlete recovering from a concussion should avoid alcohol.

If these interventions do not result in adequate sleep there are medications that may be considered. As with all medications, these should be discussed with and supervised by a physician.

A safe and common medication often used to treat insomnia is called melatonin. Melatonin is actually not a medication; it is a hormone. All of us have melatonin in our blood. It is secreted into the blood by a gland in the brain known as the pineal gland. When it gets dark, the pineal gland secretes melatonin into the bloodstream. Melatonin makes us feel sleepy. This is why we get tired when it is dark. Taking melatonin by mouth can help athletes suffering from insomnia after a concussion fall asleep.

As noted above, amitriptyline can be used to treat post-concussive insomnia, especially in athletes who are also suffering from post-concussive headaches. In addition, many other therapies and medications can be used to treat insomnia. Nonmedical therapies such as chronotherapy, psychotherapy, herbal teas, relaxation techniques, and phototherapy may be useful. Medications such as trazodone, zolpidem, other tricyclic antidepressants (besides amitriptyline), and various other medications may be helpful in certain situations. As always, it is best to discuss the options that are best for you or your athlete with an expert in the assessment and management of sport-related concussion.

Depression

Depression is common in athletes who do not recover quickly from their concussions. The most important thing you can do if you are having depression after a concussion is tell someone such as a doctor, a school nurse, a counselor, a psychologist, or another professional who can get you help. This is especially true for athletes who feel hopeless. Thoughts of harming oneself or killing oneself are particularly concerning and should be reported immediately. Fortunately, such profound depression is rare. More commonly, athletes are simply saddened by their injury, by the fact that they cannot participate in sports, and by the fact that they have more difficulty with schoolwork and other cognitive tasks. It is frustrating. Depression is understandable. But it can usually be overcome with proper treatment.

Seeing a sports psychologist can be helpful in treating depression after a sport-related concussion. Sports psychologists are trained in psychology, and have extra training in the psychological issues specifically related to sports and athletes. In addition to improving the athlete's mood and treating the depression, a sports psychologist can teach the athlete coping strategies, ways of dealing with the injury, with the cognitive dysfunction, and with the limitations imposed on activities and functioning as a result of the concussion.

As noted above, in certain circumstances, allowing athletes to return to aerobic exercise is safe. This can go a long way in improving an athlete's mood and overall disposition. This option should be discussed with the clinician managing the athlete's concussion.

Finally, sometimes these interventions are not enough, and the athlete remains depressed despite them. In such cases, medication may be considered. This option should be discussed with the athlete's doctor. Many doctors will refer an athlete to another clinician who is experienced in treating depression with medicine, as opposed to prescribing it themselves.

Cognitive Dysfunction

As noted previously, cognitive processes are those that involve thinking, reasoning, concentrating, and remembering. These processes are negatively impacted by concussion. Thinking becomes slower. Memory becomes worse. Concentration becomes difficult. This can be frustrating, especially for student athletes. As with all the signs and symptoms of concussion, these problems should resolve shortly, over the course of a few days to weeks. In some small percentage of athletes, however, these problems persist for weeks to months. Many athletes seek treatment for these problems. The best and most effective treatments are discussed above in the section on cognitive rest and academic accommodations. However, some athletes' problems will be so severe and last for so long that they negatively impact the athlete's quality of life to such an extent that the athlete seeks other treatments.

Unfortunately, there is no proven, generally accepted therapy for treating the cognitive dysfunction caused by sport-related concussion or concussive brain injuries sustained outside of sports. There are, however, some potential medications which might be considered. Some medical studies have shown that these medications can help maintain the brain function of people who have sustained a traumatic brain injury. Other studies have shown no benefit. These medications act directly on the cells of the brain, or neurons. Like all medications, there are side effects associated with them. Athletes taking them should be monitored closely. Before deciding whether or not to take one of these medications, the athlete should understand all of the potential risks and the likelihood of benefit. These medications should only be prescribed by a physician with expertise and experience in the assessment and management of concussive brain injuries.

One such medication is called amantadine. Amantadine was initially developed as an anti-influenza agent, a medication used to treat or prevent illness caused by influenza virus. But, as often happens in medicine and science, other uses were discovered serendipitously. Physicians noticed that when patients with Parkinson's disease were taking amantadine as treatment for or in order to prevent the flu, the symptoms of their Parkinson's disease improved. Thus, amantadine started to be used to treat Parkinson's disease. Later, during an influenza outbreak, intravenous amantadine was given to patients in a neurological intensive care unit, a special part of the hospital where patients with serious brain, spinal cord, or nerve-related illnesses and injuries are managed. Physicians treating these patients noticed that while they were on amantadine, patients suffering from a traumatic brain injury had some improvement in their cognitive function. This suggested that amantadine might spare the loss of some brain function in patients who have suffered from a traumatic brain injury, like concussion. Thus, studies were designed to investigate the utility of amantadine as a potential treatment for traumatic brain injury. As noted, some studies showed that it was helpful. Others showed no benefit. Some of the evidence suggests that perhaps, amantadine is more useful in treating children who have sustained traumatic brain injury than it is in treating adults with traumatic brain injury. Until further data is available, amantadine should be considered a potential agent, as opposed to a proven agent, for the treatment of concussive brain injury.

As with all medications, amantadine has some side effects. However, it is generally well tolerated. In fact, the medicine is so safe, that the current Federal Drug Administration (FDA) approval for amantadine is for use by healthy children during an influenza outbreak, in order to prevent them from getting the flu. Still, it acts directly on the cells of the brain, increasing the amount of dopamine transmitted between neurons. Amantadine cannot be stopped abruptly, as there is a risk of developing malignant hyperthermia, a medical condition that causes painful rigidity of the muscles and high fevers. There is some concern over the potential for birth defects in the children of women who are pregnant or who become pregnant while taking amantadine. Therefore, careful thought should go into the potential risks and benefits of taking amantadine when deciding whether or not it should be used to treat a concussion.

Methylphenidate is another medication that has been studied to treat cognitive dysfunction after traumatic brain injury. Many readers will be familiar with methylphenidate as a treatment for attention deficit/hyperactivity disorder (ADHD). Others will recognize some of the brand names for this medication, such as Ritalin and Concerta. Methylphenidate is the most thoroughly studied medicine for treating cognitive dysfunction after traumatic brain injury. In fact, several high-quality studies have shown that methylphenidate preserves some of the cognitive function of patients recovering from traumatic brain injury. As with all medications, there are some potential risks in taking methylphenidate. Like all medications, it has side effects. Furthermore, it can be habit forming. There is little evidence showing benefits in the cognitive performance of children taking methylphenidate after a traumatic brain injury. Therefore, some argue, it is more appropriate for older athletes than for younger athletes. As with all medications, the risks and benefits of methylphenidate should be discussed with the doctor managing your athlete's sport-related concussion.

Other medications have been investigated as potential therapies for the treatment of cognitive dysfunction after traumatic brain injury including, doenpezil, rivastigmine, cytidine diphosphoryl choline (CDP-choline), fluoxetine, sertraline, pramiracetam, bromocriptine, and atomoxetine. The evidence for these medicines is limited. Each must be carefully considered and discussed with an expert in the assessment and management of concussive brain injury prior to starting.

Cognitive rehabilitation is another potential therapy for the treatment of sport-related concussions. The Brain Injury Association of America defines cognitive rehabilitation as "a systematically applied set of medical and therapeutic services designed to improve cognitive functioning and participation in activities that may be affected by difficulties in one or more cognitive domains." Simply, it is a way of retraining the brain to perform activities that, prior to injury, it was able to perform readily. There is little evidence supporting its use after sport-related concussions. Since most athletes will recover from sport-related concussions relatively quickly, the routine use of cognitive rehabilitation after sport-related concussion is unnecessary. However, for athletes suffering from prolonged cognitive dysfunction after sustaining a sport-related concussion, cognitive rehabilitation may be considered.

In summary, the vast majority of athletes will recover from a sport-related concussion quickly, within days to weeks. Physical and cognitive rest will often

be the only therapies necessary to achieve a complete recovery from a sport-related concussion. The therapies discussed in this chapter will be unnecessary for most readers and their athletes. However, a small percentage of concussed athletes will suffer prolonged recoveries, lasting weeks to months, or even up to a year. Some athletes will have such profound symptoms that their quality of life will be negatively impacted by their injuries. For this small minority, other therapies should be considered to assist them with their recovery. The potential risks and adverse effects of these medications must be considered and weighed against the likelihood of benefit. These therapies should be tailored to address the athletes' most bothersome symptoms. Athletes engaging in these potential therapies should be closely monitored in conjunction with a clinician experienced in the assessment and management of sport-related concussions or concussive brain injuries in general.

Suggested Readings

Beers, S. R., A. Skold, C. E. Dixon, and P. D. Adelson, Neurobehavioral Effects of Amantadine after Pediatric Traumatic Brain Injury: A Preliminary Report. *J Head Trauma Rehabil*, 2005. 20: 450–63.

Chew, E., and R. D. Zafonte, Pharmacological Management of Neurobehavioral Disorders Following Traumatic Brain Injury—A State-of-the-Art Review. *J Rehabil Res Dev*, 2009. 46(6): 851–79.

Lenaerts, M. E., and J. R. Couch, Posttraumatic Headache. *Curr Treat Options Neurol*, 2004. 6: 507–17.

McCrory, P., et al., Consensus Statement on Concussion in Sport: The 3rd International Conference on Concussion in Sport Held in Zurich, November 2008. *J Athl Train*, 2009. 44(4): 434–48.

Meehan, W. P. 3rd, P. d'Hemecourt, and R. D. Comstock, High School Concussions in the 2008–2009 Academic Year: Mechanism, Symptoms, and Management. *Am J Sports Med*, 2010. 38(12): 2405–9.

Rao, V, and P. Rollings, Sleep Disturbances Following Traumatic Brain Injury. *Curr Treat Options Neurol*, 2002. 4: 77–87.

Tenovuo, O, Pharmacological Enhancement of Cognitive and Behavioral Deficits after Traumatic Brain Injury. *Curr Opin Neurol*, 2006. 19: 528–33.

Whyte, J., T. Hart, K. Schuster, M. Fleming, M. Polansky, and H. B. Coslett, Effects of Methylphenidate on Attentional Function after Traumatic Brain Injury. A Randomized, Placebo-Controlled Trial. *Am J Phys Med Rehabil*, 1997. 76: 440–50.

9

ASSESSING RECOVERY FROM CONCUSSION: WHEN IS IT SAFE FOR MY ATHLETE TO RETURN TO SPORTS?

On Sunday September 12, 2010, the Philadelphia Eagles were playing the Green Bay packers. It was the second quarter. While tackling Green Bay wide receiver Greg Jennings, the head of Eagles linebacker Stewart Bradley bounced off of the right hip of his teammate and fellow linebacker Ernie Sims. On video replay, Stewart's head was seen snapping sharply back while twisting to his right. When the play was over, Bradley struggled to stand up. After approximately seven seconds of balancing himself tenuously on all four limbs, he rose to his feet. He stumbled forward, only to fall again, face first, onto the ground. He was dazed. His fellow players knew something was wrong. Even his opponent, Green Bay's Greg Jennings, started waving the medical staff onto the field to tend to Bradley.

Stewart Bradley was concussed.

Yet later in that same quarter, Bradley was returned to play. This sparked a lot of controversy in the sports community, with sports writers and sports blog enthusiasts taking Philadelphia coach Andy Reid and the Eagles medical staff to task. According to the guidelines adopted by the National Football League less than a year earlier, a player who suffers a concussion should not return to play on the same day. The Eagles responded by saying Bradley had been able to "go through the protocol." But with the nation watching on television, it seemed that Bradley, who had clearly suffered a concussion, was returned to play during the same game.

This chapter will discuss the strategies used for monitoring an athlete's recovery over time. Concussion monitoring focuses on three main categories: 1) the recovery from symptoms, 2) the recovery of brain function, and 3) the recovery of balance and motor tasks. The determination of recovery is made by assessing these three indicators of injury. Often, after an athlete is believed to have fully recovered, an additional rest period is recommended. When an athlete is cleared to return to play, there are international guidelines through which athletes should progress, prior to participating in competition.

Some of the therapies discussed in chapters 7 and 8 may be used to help you or your athlete recover from a sport-related concussion. But how do we know when an athlete is recovered?

Three main components of recovery are monitored after an athlete sustains a concussion: symptoms, balance, and cognitive function. Ideally, there will be a baseline value for each of these components, as discussed in chapter 7. Athletes will be monitored until they return to their baseline scores. If no baseline data are available for a given athlete, then clinicians will do their best to determine when complete recovery has occurred. Often, in the absence of baseline data, a period of extra rest will be added to the recovery period, prior to clearing an athlete for contact. This extra rest period will often be longer for younger athletes. Prior to clearing an athlete to resume contact or collision play, baseline data should be collected so they may be used in the unfortunate event of future concussions.

Symptoms: As noted previously, symptoms are most often measured using a symptom inventory. An example of a commonly used symptom inventory is shown in Figure 9.1. Most athletes are given a list of symptoms, followed by a scale of severity from 0 to 6, where 0 means the athlete is not experiencing the symptom and 6 means the symptom is as severe as the athlete can imagine. The athlete is asked to circle the number that corresponds to the degree of severity for each of the symptoms listed. These numbers can then be added together in order to get a total post-concussion symptom scale score. For example, if an athlete has a pretty bad headache, some nausea, some trouble falling asleep, and decreased energy on the day he fills out the symptom inventory, his scale might look like this:

Figure 9.1
Example of Part of a Post-concussion Symptom Scale

Headache	0	1	2	3	4	(5)	6
Nausea	0	1	(2)	3	4	5	6
Difficulty sleeping	0	(1)	2	3	4	5	6
Decreased energy	0	1	2	(3)	4	5	6

If he is not experiencing any other symptoms, a "0" would be circled for the remainder of the symptoms included in the inventory.

5 for headache + 2 for nausea + 1 for difficulty sleeping
+ 3 for decreased energy = 11.

Thus, his total symptom score would be 11.

Many people will have some mild symptoms even when they are not injured. Some people have headaches and nausea from time to time. Some have difficulty falling asleep even when they are not injured or concussed. By measuring these symptoms before a concussion, clinicians can determine whether or not an athlete's symptoms are worse after their injury. Similarly, they can see how long it takes for athletes symptoms to return to their preseason, "baseline," level. By measuring all symptoms before the start of the season, athletes who were having some symptoms before their concussion won't mistakenly be considered concussed after they have recovered, even if they are still experiencing the same headaches, nausea, decreased energy, or difficulty sleeping they were having before their injury. For athletes who have no symptoms when they are in their usual state of health, their initial, preseason, baseline symptoms inventory score will be 0.

One can imagine, however, some athletes will show up for their preseason assessment after they were up late at night studying. Or, on the day of their preseason baseline measurement, they might have a cold or the flu. Thus, they may have many symptoms when they complete their "baseline" symptom inventory that are not "baseline" at all. They are due to the fact that the athlete just happens to be tired or ill on the day the inventory is taken. Thus, another approach is to only measure those symptoms that are due to a concussion. When performed this way, every athlete should score a 0 at the start of the season (unless they are recovering from a concussion from a prior season). When the baseline symptom inventory is completed in this way, athletes who sustain a concussion should be asked to complete follow-up symptom inventories after injury by circling *only those symptoms that started at the time of their concussion and have not yet gone away.*

Both approaches to symptom inventories are reasonable. Whichever method is used, no athlete should be returned to play until the symptoms due to his or her concussion have completely resolved. That means, using the first method noted above, no athlete should be returned to play until his or her baseline symptom inventory score is equal to what it was prior to the start of the season. Using the second method described above, no athlete should return to play until his or her symptom score is equal to zero. Although reasonable exceptions to this rule may sometimes be made, they should be infrequent and supervised by a clinician with expertise in the assessment and management of sport-related concussion.

Medications are often used to help treat the symptoms of an athlete who experiences a prolonged recovery from a sport-related concussion. Once the athlete is no longer experiencing these symptoms, medications should be discontinued. Some medications however cannot be stopped abruptly. Therefore, even though the athlete may no longer be experiencing symptoms from his or her concussion, the physician prescribing a medication will recommend the athlete continues to take it for some period of time. Often the medication will have to be tapered as opposed to abruptly stopped. When tapering off of a medication, an athlete decreases the daily dose slowly, over a period of days to weeks, until he or she is on such a small dose that it can be stopped safely. In order to be returned to sports safely, athletes must remain symptom-free even after the medication has been stopped. Therefore, athletes who are still taking a medication to treat the signs and symptoms of concussion should not be returned to sports, even if they are symptom-free while on the medication. Exceptions to this rule, as always, should be made by clinicians with experience in the assessment and management of sport-related concussion.

Headaches are the most common symptom of sport-related concussion. There is even some evidence that athletes who sustain migraine-like symptoms after concussion take longer to recover than other athletes. Recent medical investigations are considering whether or not athletes who have family members who suffer migraine headaches also take longer to recover from sport-related concussions than other athletes. These associations between migraine headaches and recovery from concussion have led some clinicians to believe that certain people, who may be predisposed to migraine headaches may also be predisposed to suffering sport-related concussions.

We all suffer headaches from time to time. Some people have very specific headaches that they suffer on a fairly regular basis. Many readers will know someone who suffers from migraine headaches. It is well known that trauma to the head can result in the onset of migraine headaches, even when the patient has not sustained a concussion, or when the patient has recovered from his or her concussion. Therefore, it can sometimes be unclear whether athletes are experiencing headaches because they are still recovering from their concussions, or whether they have headaches that were brought about by their trauma, despite the fact that they have recovered from their concussions. Again, decisions about when an athlete should return to sport should be made by a clinician with expertise in the assessment and management of sport-related concussion.

As noted, many of the signs and symptoms of sport-related concussion can be seen in other illnesses or disease processes. The treatment of a sport-related concussion in and of itself can result in some symptoms. Sport-related concussions can result in irritability, depressed mood, low energy, and insomnia. However, the same symptoms can result from the treatment of sport-related concussions, namely, physical and cognitive rest. Most athletes choose to participate in sports. Most of them enjoy playing sports. They enjoy exercising. Exercise improves their mood and overall sense of well-being. Since one of the treatments of sport-related concussions is physical rest, these athletes are removed from sports and exercise during their recovery. This often results in the onset of irritability, depression, and increased emotionality. Therefore, it can be difficult to determine, at times, whether or not the symptoms are due to incomplete recovery from a sport-related concussion or due to the treatment of sport-related concussion. In order to help distinguish between these two possibilities, doctors will occasionally allow an athlete to return to some safe, light aerobic activity prior to full resolution of his or her symptoms. Often, being allowed to exercise in such a manner will improve the patient's mood, as well as alleviate depression, help with difficulty sleeping, and decrease their irritability.

Regular exercise can also increase one's energy. Therefore, being removed from exercise can decrease one's energy. People who lead a sedentary lifestyle often complain of feeling fatigued, tired, and having low energy. Regular exercise can improve these symptoms. Again, since athletes have been removed from exercise and physical activity during the recovery from sport-related concussions, decreased energy may result. Returning to some light aerobic activity in a safe setting can often improve their overall energy and help distinguish between incomplete recovery from sport-related concussion and the negative side effects of physical rest.

While exercise can improve one's overall energy during the waking hours, physical exertion is also tiring. Therefore, many athletes will sleep well through the night, often requiring more hours of sleep then sedentary individuals. Once again, the removal from physical exertion as part of treatment for a sport-related concussion can result in sleep disturbance or insomnia. Insomnia, however, is one of the main symptoms of concussion. In particular, athletes who take longer than days to weeks to recover from their concussion will rank insomnia as one of their most significant symptoms. By allowing athletes to return to some light aerobic activity in a safe setting, their sleep can be improved.

In addition to the symptoms an athlete reports, an athlete's signs, including balance, are also used to track his or her recovery and to determine when it is safe to return to sports. As noted, many athletes will have a balance error system score recorded prior to the start of the season. After a concussion, athletes' balance is often worse. It improves as they recover, until they are just as steady on their feet as they were before the season started. An athlete should not be considered completely recovered until his or her balance has returned to preinjury levels.

Again, some exceptions to this rule may be made. One can imagine athletes might sustain an ankle or knee injury at the same time as their concussions. They may recover from their concussions quite quickly. However, they may still have some residual injury to the ankle or knee. This may adversely affect their balance. Decisions to return athletes to play prior to full recovery of their preseason balance should be made by a clinician with expertise in the assessment and management of sport-related concussion.

Brain function is also used to assess recovery from a sport-related concussion. Most commonly the assessment of brain function is measured using computerized neuropsychological testing as discussed in previous chapters. Ideally, athletes will have measurements of their brain function prior to the start of the athletic season. In the event of a concussion, their brain function will be reassessed and compared to what it was prior to their injury. Any deficits from their preseason or baseline functioning should be considered reflective of injury. Athletes should not be returned to sport until their brain function has recovered back to its pre-injury level.

The assessment of these neuropsychological scores can be somewhat complicated. Any time people take a test of any kind more than once, they are likely to
get a different score than they did previously. People often do a little bit better
or little bit worse than they did before. This is expected. Therefore, athletic
trainers, doctors, neuropsychologists, and other people interpreting these computerized neuropsychological tests must take this normal background variation
in scores into account. They must decide when a test score is so much better or
so much worse than a previous test score that it reflects true injury or true
recovery as opposed to simply background variability. Methods of statistical
analysis are used to assist in this determination.

Furthermore, performance on these computerized neuropsychological tests
can be affected by many factors. If athletes are ill at the time of the test, they
may perform worse than if they were healthy. Similarly, if they are tired at the
time of the test, they will perform worse than when they are well rested. Athletes who are depressed may perform more poorly than they would if they were
in good spirits. In addition, athletes will have different motivation. Those taking
a preseason baseline test may not be motivated to do well, since there's nothing
at stake. An athlete taking a post-injury test 10 days before a championship
game, however, may be highly motivated to score well on the test. Likewise,
some athletes may be participating in a sport that they do not particularly like.
They may have little desire to return to that sport and therefore be less motivated when taking tests after injury than they would be if they enjoyed their
sport. All of these factors must be taken into account by the clinician who is
interpreting the scores.

As computerized neuropsychological tests become more common in the
assessment and management of sport-related concussions, athletes become
more familiar with the process and how these tests are used. Therefore, some
athletes will intentionally do poorly on their preseason baseline. That way, if
they sustain a sport-related concussion during the season, they might still be
able to achieve their baseline scores, even while concussed. In this way, these
athletes hope to be returned to sport prior to full recovery. They should be cau-
tioned, however, that many of these computer programs have hidden mecha-
nisms within the test that allow clinicians to determine whether or not the
athlete put forth a good effort. Experienced clinicians will be able to decipher
whether or not an athlete has purposefully performed poorly. Those athletes
will be required to repeat the test prior to being cleared for game play.

Athletes should not be cleared to resume sports until they have reachieved
their prior levels of brain function. Again some exceptions to this rule may be
considered. Rarely, athletes may have the day of their lives when they take their
baseline test. They may score much higher than they would on any other occasion. Therefore, some athletes who have had complete resolution of their symptoms, who have had complete return of their balance, and who remain
symptom-free despite days or weeks of full participation in the noncontact
activities of their respective sports may be cleared to return to play despite not

having reachieved their preinjury neuropsychological test scores. Again, decisions such as this should be made by clinicians with expertise in the assessment and management of sport-related concussion.

Recently, there has been some debate in the medical and neuropsychological literature regarding who should be interpreting these scores. Some feel that these computerized assessments should only be interpreted by a neuropsychologist. Others argue that these assessments are a relatively small part of neuropsychology, and other clinicians with different medical backgrounds can be taught to administer and interpret these scores reliably. As many concerned athletes, coaches, and parents may hear this debate, I will offer my opinion and some clarification.

As a medical doctor I was trained to do many things. One of those things was to perform a physical examination of the patient. There are various components of the physical examination. The component of the physical examination that relates to the brain, the nerves, and the ability of brain function is known as the neurological examination. While learning the neurological examination, medical students are taught how the normal body appears, how it reacts to certain stimuli, and how the ill or injured body reacts differently than the normal, healthy body. For example, many readers will recall a time when they were seen by a doctor and had a light shone in their eyes. The black circle in the center of people's eyes is known as the pupil. Light travels through the pupil to a nerve at the back of the eye that is connected to the brain. This is how we are able to see. The brain interprets the light that strikes this nerve at the back of the eye. When a bright light is shined into the eye of a normal, healthy patient, the pupil will become smaller, or constrict. In certain disease processes or other states the pupil is abnormally small and will not constrict. In other disease processes the pupil is abnormally large and will not constrict. Sometimes the pupil of the left eye is a different size than the pupil of the right eye. This can be due to disease or injury. But it can also be a normal finding.

Doctors have learned how to interpret these findings and determine whether or not they are normal, due to disease, or due to injury. This is one small part of the neurological examination. And the neurological examination is one small part of the overall physical examination. And the physical examination is a small part of what the doctor learns while going through medical school. While I do not think it is possible for someone to learn everything that is taught during medical education without going to medical school and completing a residency, I do believe that other clinicians can be taught to perform a neurological examination properly. Indeed, nurses, nurse practitioners, physician assistants, and neuropsychologists themselves can be taught certain components of the neurological examination.

Likewise, physicians, athletic trainers, nurses, and other medical personnel can be taught to administer and interpret computerized neuropsychological tests without having to complete the full training of a neuropsychologist. Certainly, there will be times when these computerized neuropsychological assessments will be difficult to interpret. At times like this, the opinion of a neuropsychologist should be sought. Indeed, where I work at the Sports Concussion Clinic in the Division of Sports Medicine at Children's Hospital Boston, we work very closely with many neuropsychologists on interpreting these scores. In addition, our neuropsychologists help us make the diagnosis of concussion, help determine when an athlete has recovered from a concussion, and provide academic planning for students who have significant brain dysfunction after sustaining a sport-related concussion. Neuropsychologists are an essential part of our sports concussion clinic.

The best approach for managing concussive brain injuries involves a team of personnel, including all of the various specialties and subspecialties mentioned in this book. However, not all athletic teams, hospitals, or medical clinics will have access to neuropsychologists. There are relatively few neuropsychologists in comparison to the number of athletic trainers, physicians, nurses, and other medical professionals combined. Therefore, other medical professionals should be taught to administer and interpret computerized neuropsychological test scores for the limited purpose of assessing sport-related concussions and determining when an athlete has recovered.

Furthermore, many neuropsychologists who are well versed in the traditional types of neuropsychological testing will not be familiar with the computerized neuropsychological tests used for assessing sport-related concussions. Specific training on administering and interpreting computerized tests is necessary, even for neuropsychologists who trained only in the more traditional paradigms.

To ensure the highest quality of care is given to all athletes, other medical professionals need to be trained to administer and interpret computerized neuropsychological tests for the limited function of assessing sport-related concussions. Ideally, this would be in conjunction with a trained neuropsychologist to whom patients could then be referred for more in-depth analyses when necessary.

While symptoms, balance, and neurocognitive function are the three main components in helping determine when an athlete has recovered from a sport-related concussion, there are many other factors that are considered before returning an athlete to sport. Even when an athlete has recovered fully from a sport-related concussion, medical professionals may recommend further avoidance of high-risk athletic activities for a period of time. Some of the other factors used to determine when an athlete can return to sports are discussed below.

NUMBER OF LIFETIME CONCUSSIONS

Although there is no absolute number of concussions after which an athlete should not return to contact sports, collision sports, or other high-risk athletic activities, most clinicians still take the total number of concussions an athlete has sustained during his or her lifetime into consideration when making decisions about an athlete's return to sports. In general a more conservative approach is warranted with an athlete who has sustained several concussions as compared to an athlete who has sustained only one or two. In other words, athletes who have sustained multiple concussions should be given more time to recover from their injuries before being returned to game play or other risky activities than athletes who have only sustained one concussion.

Duration of Recovery Time from Concussion

As noted, many athletes will have full resolution of their post-concussion symptoms within a few days to weeks. In a study published in the *Journal of the American Medical Association* in 2003, 90 percent of college football players who sustained a sport-related concussion had resolution of their symptoms within 10 days. A study published in the *American Journal of Sports Medicine* in 2010 showed that nearly 85 percent of high school athletes who sustained a sport-related concussion had complete resolution of their symptoms and were deemed recovered by their athletic trainer within seven days after injury. Within one month after their injury, 98.5 percent of high school athletes who sustained a sport-related concussion were deemed recovered by their athletic trainer. However, some unfortunate minority of athletes will have symptoms that last much longer. In the Sports Concussion Clinic at Children's Hospital Boston, we have seen patients whose post-concussion symptoms and cognitive dysfunction have persisted for several months. A small handful of athletes have taken a year or longer to completely recover from their concussions. Athletes who experience these prolonged recoveries are often held out of contact sports, collision sports, or other risky athletic activities for a longer period of time than those who recover more quickly. This is to allow the brain further time to heal before exposing it to another potential injury.

Amount of Force Resulting in Concussions

We have all seen major collisions in American football or ice hockey that have resulted in an athlete suffering a sport-related concussion. However for some athletes, especially if they have sustained prior sport-related concussions, a much lower level of force results in a concussive brain injury. If an athlete appears to be sustaining concussions with a progressively lower level of force, clinicians become concerned. Often, we will recommend a longer period of recovery even after symptoms resolve, balance is returned to normal, and brain function has recovered to baseline, before clearing such an athlete to return to their sport.

Type of Activity or Sport to Which the Athlete Wishes to Return

The type of activity or sport to which the athlete wishes to return is a key component in deciding when they may return. Tennis is a relatively low-risk sport as far as sport-related concussion is concerned. Therefore, an athlete might be returned to tennis almost as soon as he or she has recovered from a concussion. If that same athlete, however, wished to return to ice hockey, football, or rugby, clinicians would often recommend a longer waiting period. In some cases not only the sport the athlete wishes to play but also the position the athlete will be playing factors into decisions regarding return to play. For example, some clinicians will require a longer period of recovery for cheerleaders who are flyers, given the high-risk nature of their cheerleading activities, compared to other cheerleaders.

THE GOALS OF THE ATHLETE

Athletes' long-term goals play a major role in determining if and when they return to their sport. It is not uncommon for athletes who have sustained three or four concussions over the course of their lifetime to wish to return to their contact or collision sport. Those of us practicing medicine know that there is a risk of losing cognitive function after sustaining multiple concussions. The exact number of concussions that results in a permanent loss of cognitive function is unknown. In fact, it is likely that there is no exact number. It is more likely that the number is different for each athlete, depending on the physical and biological characteristics of the athlete, the forces involved in each injury, and many other factors that we in medicine have not yet elucidated. Some athletes will sustain many concussions and not suffer permanent losses of cognitive function. How long an athlete must wait before returning to sport after a concussion, or whether or not they should return to sport at all after sustaining multiple concussions, depends on their lifetime goals. If a junior in college who plays for the varsity team has sustained his fourth lifetime concussion, and his long-term goal in life is to become a veterinarian, he and his clinician may decide that the potential long-term risks of returning to sport and possibly sustaining a fifth lifetime concussion are not worth taking. However, if that same college junior plays for a high-level college program, aspires to play professional hockey in the National Hockey League, and given his current skill level, abilities, and reputation this is a realistic possibility for him, he and his clinician may decide that he will return to sport and assume the potential risks of a fifth lifetime concussion.

Although some readers may see this as controversial, it is difficult to take away somebody's livelihood, his means of earning a living, over a potential risk that may or may not ever occur. Many athletes may sustain five, six, seven, or more of concussions over the course of their lifetime without suffering permanent cognitive deficits. Others may have long-term cognitive deficits and other problems as a result of only three or four concussions. Since those of us in medicine cannot accurately predict which number of concussions will lead to long-term problems, nor which athletes are at risk for these problems, each case must be decided individually with the aspirations, concerns, and understanding of the athlete in mind. Many times, conversations about such topics will also involve all of the clinicians caring for the athlete, the athlete's loved ones, and the other important people in the athlete's life. Most often, the conversation takes place over a series of visits, lasting anywhere from several weeks to months or even years in some athletes who sustain multiple concussions over the course of their academic and professional careers.

THE SEVERITY OF COGNITIVE DEFICITS OBSERVED AFTER CONCUSSION

As we have seen, some athletes will not sustain measurable cognitive deficits in their brain function with their concussions. Other athletes will sustain mild deficits in their brain function with their sport-related concussions. Still other athletes will sustain marked and significant deficits in their brain function with their concussions. It is not uncommon for clinicians to recommend a longer time away from contact sports, collision sports, or other risky athletic activities for athletes who have sustained more dramatic deficits in their brain function after injury. For athletes who used to suffer relatively mild cognitive deficits with their first few concussions, but are now suffering much more significant cognitive deficits after sustaining multiple concussions, the length of time prior to returning to contact or collision sports is often increased to allow for further recovery.

THE SEVERITY OF SYMPTOMS EXPERIENCED BY THE ATHLETE AFTER CONCUSSION

Some athletes will experience severe, even incapacitating symptoms as a result of their concussions. Most clinicians will recommend longer times away from sport for those athletes who have experienced more severe symptoms than for those who have only mild symptoms after their concussion. In addition, if athletes who complained of relatively mild symptoms after their first concussion now have more significant symptoms after sustaining multiple concussions, clinicians often recommend longer recovery times.

THE AGE OF THE ATHLETE

Concussion is one of the few injuries from which it seems adults recover more quickly than children. Medical studies conducted in older athletes have shown shorter recovery times after sport-related concussions than medical studies conducted in younger athletes. The reason for this is unclear. It could be that the younger, developing brain of pediatric athletes heals more slowly than the fully developed brain of more mature athletes. It could also be, however, that those athletes who require long times in order to recover from their sport-related concussions stop playing high-risk sports at a younger age. Thus, they are no longer at risk of sustaining a sport-related concussion. Until we know more about the recovery from a sport-related concussion and how recovery is affected by age, it is prudent to keep the pediatric athlete out of sports for a longer period of time than the older athlete.

Furthermore, older athletes are more likely to play for a team with greater resources. Younger athletes often compete for teams that have no athletic trainer, no team physician, no emergency action plan, and no concussion protocol. These athletes have fewer baseline assessments available to help determine when they are recovered. Since it is often more difficult to determine when these athletes are fully recovered, longer recovery time is frequently recommended.

OTHER FACTORS

Many other factors may contribute to the decision to return an athlete to participation in sports. These decisions are complicated. Since the medical community has only recently begun to pay attention to sport-related concussions, there is much we do not know about them. No specific tests are available to definitively diagnose sport-related concussions or determine precisely when recovery has occurred. While it is now known that some athletes will suffer long-term effects from sustaining multiple sport-related concussions, we do not yet have the ability to predict which athletes are vulnerable to these long-term effects, how many injuries are needed before one suffers these long-term effects, or what other factors might help predict which athletes are likely to develop these long-term problems. Until such information is available, doctors, athletes, parents, neuropsychologists, and all others involved in the assessment and management of sport-related concussions must weigh the potential risks and benefits of each individual case prior to determining when it is safe for an athlete to return to contact sports, collision sports, or other risky athletic activities.

In summary, clinicians use athletes' symptoms, balance, and cognitive function to help determine when it is safe to return to sports after sustaining a sport-related concussion. Ideally, measurements of these factors are taken before the athlete sustains a concussion. When such data are available, most athletes should not be returned to sports until after they have re-achieved their baseline levels. In the absence of such baseline measurements, longer recovery times are often recommended. Similarly, longer recovery times are recommended for younger athletes, athletes who have sustained multiple concussions, athletes with pronounced signs and symptoms after their concussions, athletes who sustain concussions after collisions involving minimal force, athletes with prolonged recoveries, as well as athletes with other concerning circumstances. In most cases, athletes should be off of any medication used to treat their post-concussion symptoms prior to being cleared for contact or collision. Since there is no medical test available to accurately determine when it is safe for an athlete to return to contact or collision sports after a sport-related concussion, clinicians use many factors to help estimate the appropriate timetable for athletes' resumption of such activities.

Suggested Readings

Guskiewicz, K. M., et al., Cumulative Effects Associated with Recurrent Concussion in Collegiate Football Players: The NCAA Concussion Study. *JAMA*, 2003. 290(19): 2549–55.

Lau, B., et al., Neurocognitive and Symptom Predictors of Recovery in High School Athletes. *Clin J Sport Med*, 2009. 19(3): 16–21.

McCrory, P., et al., Consensus Statement on Concussion in Sport: The 3rd International Conference on Concussion in Sport Held in Zurich, November 2008. *J Athl Train*, 2009. 44(4): 434–48.

Meehan, W. P., 3rd, P. d'Hemecourt, and R. D. Comstock, High School Concussions in the 2008–2009 Academic Year: Mechanism, Symptoms, and Management. *Am J Sports Med*, 2010. 38(12): 2405–9.

10

PREVENTION: IS THERE A WAY TO PREVENT MY ATHLETE FROM SUSTAINING A CONCUSSION?

Heavyweight boxer "Iron" Mike Tyson was a veritable wrecking machine. I remember arguing with other kids in the neighborhood about whether or not we could live through an unobstructed punch from Mike Tyson. I still don't know the answer. And I don't ever want to find out.

On November 22, 1986, Mike Tyson defeated Trevor Berbick to become the youngest champion to ever win the heavyweight title. He was only 20 years old. Berbick, the heavyweight champion at the time, was well known as the last man to fight Muhammad Ali. On paper, the fight appeared fairly well matched. In fact, given his height and reach, Berbick appeared to have a slight advantage. Tyson weighed in at 221 pounds to Berbick's 218. Berbick was three inches taller at 6 feet 2 inches compared to Tyson's 5 feet 11 inches. This translated to Berbick having a significant advantage in reach. While Tyson was younger, Berbick was more mature, at 32 years old. But, as the fight would prove, this was not an even match.

During the first round, Tyson struck Berbick in the head with several powerful blows. With 23 seconds remaining in the first round, Berbick stumbled after sustaining a hard right to the head. Tyson pounced. He landed several additional blows that caused Berbick to drop his hands, clearly stunned by the assault. He was overpowered by Tyson. But he managed to remain on his feet until the bell rang. Within the first few seconds of round two, Tyson landed a series of powerful right and left hooks that knocked Berbick to the canvas.

The round continued. To those of us watching, it appeared that Berbick was simply trying to remain on his feet and survive the periodic bursts of power from the challenger. With 38 seconds left, Tyson landed a right to the body, then an uppercut to the head followed by a left hook that knocked Berbick to the canvas. Berbick tried to stand a total of three times. But he could only stumble and fall back to the canvas. He was dazed, confused, disoriented.

Trevor Berbick was concussed.

With boxers constantly at risk for sustaining concussions, it would be wonderful if there were some effective means of preventing a concussion.

This chapter will present potential ways of preventing concussions in athletes. The theories behind individual prevention strategies will be reviewed. Strategies used by larger athletic organizations will be discussed. The evidence against or in support of these strategies, when available, will be included.

Unfortunately, there is no scientific, medically proven way of preventing a concussion. As discussed previously, there are no helmets or mouth guards that are medically proven to reduce an athlete's risk of concussion. However, the experience of experts in the assessment and management of athletes has led to several strategies that are likely to help reduce the risk of sustaining a sport-related concussion, the recovery time after a sport-related concussion, and the risk of suffering long-term injury after sport-related concussions.

EDUCATION

There are many ways that education can reduce the risk of sustaining a sport-related concussion, as well as the risk of suffering long-term effects after sport-related concussions. First, it is thought that the risk of sustaining a sport-related concussion is higher after a recent concussion. This comes from studies conducted in college-aged American football players. One such study reported that athletes who sustained two concussions in the same season suffered their injuries within 10 days of each other. Therefore, educating athletes, coaches, and parents to avoid returning an athlete to play too soon can reduce the risk of these second injuries. Similarly, we have already learned that an athlete will recover more quickly from a concussion by avoiding vigorous physical activity and vigorous cognitive activity. By educating athletes, coaches, and parents about the need for physical and cognitive rest during recovery, we can reduce the duration of time an athlete experiences symptoms and reduce the overall intensity of an athlete's symptoms while he or she is recovering from a sport-related concussion.

Additionally, the risks of suffering long-term problems after sport-related concussions increases as the number of concussions sustained over an athletic career increases. By learning more about the potential long-term effects of sport-related concussions, we hope that athletes will be more likely to report their injuries, manage their injuries appropriately, and refrain from returning to play prematurely. In fact, a medical study published in the journal *Injury Prevention* in 2003 showed that athletes who undergo a concussion education program learn more about concussion, and even learn to change their actions by avoiding certain penalties after the concussion training.

For example, a concussion is more likely to occur when an athlete does not see a hit coming. Certain types of hits are more likely to result in a concussion than others. Educating athletes to avoid these types of hits can reduce the number of concussions. One such way of educating athletes has been studied in youth ice hockey. As part of this effort, players are given talks, brochures, and watch an educational video about hitting from behind. Because a hockey player cannot see a hit that is coming from behind, this is a high-risk situation as far as sport-related concussion is concerned. In order to reduce hits from behind, one league has even placed an octagonal red stop sign on the back of player's jerseys to remind their opponents not to strike them from the back.

Also included under the heading of education should be the teaching of proper technique. Purposeful heading in soccer is a commonly debated topic that can help illustrate the importance of teaching proper technique. As noted earlier in the text, although there is no medical or scientific data to support the hypothesis that purposeful heading in soccer causes sport-related concussions, many people contend that this is true. In response to this possibility, some soccer organizations have disallowed athletes who are less than 10 years old to engage in purposeful heading of the soccer ball. I believe that this approach does more harm than good. I would recommend that younger athletes use smaller and softer soccer balls. Since they are not as capable as their older counterparts of generating high velocities when throwing or kicking a soccer ball, these athletes can learn the proper skills and techniques of heading a soccer ball at a younger age while avoiding high risk exposure to potential injury.

Heading a soccer ball requires timing. It requires leg, back, and neck muscle strength. It requires physical coordination. It requires coordination between the eyes watching the soccer ball approach and the muscles of the legs, back, abdomen, and neck used for purposefully heading the soccer ball. These skills are best developed at younger ages, when athletes can only generate a certain amount of momentum with their kicks and throw-ins. I do not think the first time an athlete attempts to purposefully head the ball should be when it is drilled in the air with the force that some older children are capable of generating—say, after it is kicked 30 feet in the air and 40 yards downfield by a powerful and skilled 10- or 11-year-old goalkeeper.

HEADS-UP PLAYING

Playing with the head up, constantly being aware of what is taking place around one, can reduce the number of unexpected body checks the athlete experiences. Since most concussions occur when an athlete does not see the hit coming, keeping the head up and being aware can potentially reduce the risk of sustaining a concussion. When athletes see a hit coming, they are able to brace themselves for impact and absorb the force of impact in such a way that their risk of injury is reduced. Medical studies, again in youth ice hockey, have shown that players who see a hit coming and are able to absorb the hit properly are less likely to suffer a sport-related concussion. A study published in the medical journal *Pediatrics* in 2010 showed that in adolescent ice hockey players, collisions following an anticipated hit resulted in fewer severe head impacts than collisions following unanticipated hits.

Neck Muscle Strength

Strengthening of the neck muscles may reduce an athlete's risk of sustaining concussions. Although many readers will be pleased to have put physics behind them after graduating from high school or college, a brief refresher in a simple, fundamental concept of physics will go a long way in explaining why this is. As we have already learned, athletes sustain concussions after a force is applied to their head or after a force is transmitted to their head from a blow sustained somewhere else on the body. This force results in a spinning, or rotational acceleration, of the brain. It is this rotational acceleration that causes the concussion.

Some readers may recall from physics that, mathematically, force is equal to mass multiplied by acceleration. That is to say that, when a given force is applied to an object, how quickly that object accelerates away from the force depends on its mass. This is often represented by the equation:

$$F = ma$$

where "F" represents the force of the collision, "m" represents the mass of the object, and "a" represents the acceleration of the object after impact. Although it can sound confusing when put into scientific or mathematical terms, this concept is a matter of common sense for most readers. Suppose, for example, that I were to punch a ball as hard as I could. In scientific terms, we would say I am applying a force to the ball. After the punch, the ball would roll away from me. How rapidly it accelerates away from me would depend on the mass of the ball. If I were to punch a tennis ball, it would accelerate very rapidly away from me. If, however, I were to punch a bowling ball, it would accelerate relatively slowly away from me. This is what is meant by the mathematical equation F=ma. When the same force is applied to a ball, such as by punching it, a ball with a lot of mass, such as a bowling ball, will accelerate slowly, whereas a ball with little mass, such as a tennis ball, will accelerate more rapidly.

Since it is the acceleration of the brain after a force is applied or transmitted to the head that results in a concussion, we can reduce the risk of sustaining a concussion by reducing acceleration. One way to reduce the acceleration after a given force has been applied is to increase the mass of the head. An athlete can effectively do this by flexing his or her neck muscles. The mass of the human head is approximately 5 kilograms (11 pounds). The average mass of a male adult athlete's body is approximately 85 kilograms (187 pounds). When an athlete does not see a blow to the head coming, the 5 kilograms of the head will accelerate very rapidly. If, however, athletes see the hit coming and instinctively flex their neck muscles, the head becomes rigidly attached to the body. Therefore, after the blow is delivered, the head and remainder of the body act as one unit. Instead of the 5 kilograms of the head accelerating away very rapidly, the 85 kilograms of the body accelerates away more slowly. By strengthening their neck muscles, athletes can attach their heads to their body, so to speak, more effectively. This will reduce the acceleration of the head after impact and thereby reduce the risk of sustaining sport-related concussions.

Athletes can add the following simple strengthening exercises to their current resistance training in an effort to reduce their risk of sport-related concussions. As with all resistance training, particularly in pediatric athletes, emphasis should be placed on a proper and safe technique. Pediatric athletes who are unfamiliar with resistance training should be coached and supervised by an adult with expertise in resistance training of the pediatric athlete. The below descriptions are solely for the purpose of describing the exercises available to the reader. Anyone planning to engage in these exercises should consult a proper manual or seek professional assistance.

1. Shrugs. A common resistance exercise that will be familiar to many readers. They can be performed using either a barbell or dumbbells. Perhaps the easiest way to do shrugs is for the athlete to have a dumbbell of appropriate weight in each hand. The arms are extended at the side. The athlete raises his or her shoulders lifting the weight of the dumbbell, and then slowly relaxes to the starting position.
2. Dumbbell press. For the dumbbell press, the athlete has his or her arms raised so that the elbow is even with the shoulder on either side. The elbow is flexed to approximately 90 degrees. From this starting position, the athlete raises the dumbbell toward the ceiling while straightening the elbow. Then, the dumbbell is returned to the starting position.
3. Lateral, forward, backward, and rotational resistance exercises of the neck. Athletes playing for teams with significant resources will often have a machine that is designed to help them strengthen the muscles of their neck. However, there are some very simple resistance exercises that athletes without such resources may still perform. These resistance exercises are perhaps the easiest and one of the most effective ways of strengthening the neck muscles.

   In order to perform lateral resistance exercises, an athlete places his or her right hand along the right side of the head. The muscles of the neck are flexed such that the right ear attempts to move down toward the right shoulder. However, since the athlete is resisting this action, there is no actual movement of the head. The athlete should hold this position in active resistance for approximately 5–10 seconds. The exercise can then be performed on the left side of the head, front of the head, and back of the head. These exercises are known as the lateral, forward, and backward resistance exercises.

The rotational resistance exercises are similar. In order to perform this exercise the athlete would place his or her hand against the side of the forehead. The athlete then attempts to rotate the head toward the right or the left as when nodding "no." This motion is resisted by the hand. So there is no actual movement of the head. Again, the athlete would hold for a 5- or 10-second count and then repeat in the opposite direction.

GENERAL CONDITIONING AND STRENGTH

The stronger and faster an athlete is, the less likely the risk of injury. This is not only true for the concussion but for all types of sports injuries. It will not be too difficult for the reader to imagine that a smaller, weaker, poorly conditioned athlete is at higher risk for injury than a bigger, stronger, faster athlete. The ability to dodge a blow from one's opponent or properly absorb a blow from one's opponent will decrease the risk of sport-related concussion. These abilities come with strength, conditioning, and agility as well as practice and experience.

CONFIDENCE

In addition to being recovered from a sport-related concussion, athletes should be confident that it is time for them to return to sport. They should be without fear. This is especially true for collision sports. There are few easier ways for an athlete to become injured than to be timid or hesitant. Opponents can tell when an athlete is timid. Any slightest hesitation will serve as an opportunity to deliver a controlling blow. An athlete who is worried about sustaining another injury and is afraid while on the field or ice does not have his or her head in the game. When your head is not in the game, you're more likely to be injured. Therefore, after athletes have recovered from sport-related concussions, emphasis should focus on retraining them and getting them ready for the demands of their sport before returning them to play. When athletes return to play after sport-related concussions, they should be fast, agile, and strong. They should have no fear. They should have no concerns. They should be confident.

PADDING AND EQUIPMENT

Many concussions, particularly in pediatric sports, occur after a collision between the player and an object, such as the goalpost in football. Proper padding around such structural objects may reduce the amount of force delivered at the time of these impacts and thereby reduce the risk of sport-related concussions. Similarly, age-appropriate equipment may reduce the risk of sport-related concussions. A common example of this can be seen in soccer. Often, younger athletes are seen playing soccer using an adult, regulation-sized soccer ball. Given the small mass of the pediatric athlete's head and body compared to that of an adult, the mass of the soccer ball used in play should be reduced.

ENFORCING THE RULES OF THE GAME AND
DISCOURAGING DANGEROUS PLAY

While perhaps not always intentional, many concussions occur as a result of dangerous or illegal play. Body checks from behind in ice hockey, spear tackling to the helmet in football, dangerous kicks in soccer, elbows to the head in basketball can all result in a concussion. In fact, some medical studies conducted in junior league professional ice hockey have shown that many concussions result from illegal play. Unfortunately, this illegal play is not always noted by the referees. In addition to the general education provided in this text, consistent and diligent enforcement of the rules and regulations of the game may be one of the most effective ways of reducing the risk of sport-related concussions.

In summary, there are few medically proven ways of reducing an athlete's risk of sport-related concussion. However, educating athletes about the risks of dangerous play and the risks of returning to play before full recovery from a concussion may reduce the number of injuries and long-term consequences. Playing with the head up and being aware of one's surrounding may help prevent sport-related concussions. Athletes should not be returned to play until they are confident and ready to return to play with their "head in the game." General strengthening, conditioning, and the strengthening of an athlete's neck muscles may help decrease his or her chance of sustaining a sport-related concussion. Attention to proper placement, padding, and securing of goalposts, netting, and other structures on the surface of play may reduce the risk of concussive brain injury. Proper rule enforcement can change athlete behavior, and result in a safer environment.

SUGGESTED READINGS

Cook, D. J., et al., Evaluation of the ThinkFirst Canada, Smart Hockey, Brain and Spinal Cord Injury Prevention Video. *Inj Prev*, 2003. 9(4): 361–66.

Guskiewicz, K. M., et al., Cumulative Effects Associated with Recurrent Concussion in Collegiate Football Players: The NCAA Concussion Study. *JAMA*, 2003. 290(19): 2549–55.

Mihalik, J. P., et al., Collision Type and Player Anticipation Affect Head Impact Severity Among Youth Ice Hockey Players. *Pediatrics*, 2010. 125(6): 1394–401.

Patlak, M., and J. E. Joy, *Is Soccer Bad for Children's Heads?: Summary of the IOM Workshop on Neuropsychological Consequences of Head Impact in Youth Soccer, in The IOM Workshop on Neuropsychological Consequences of Head Impact in Youth Soccer.* 2002, National Academy of Sciences: Washington D.C.

Shewchenko, N., et al., Heading in Football. Part 2: Biomechanics of Ball Heading and Head Response. *Br J Sports Med*, 2005. 39(Suppl 1): 26–32.

Shewchenko, N., et al., Heading in Football. Part 3: Effect of Ball Properties on Head Response. *Br J Sports Med*, 2005. 39(Suppl 1): 33–39.

Viano, D. C., I. R. Casson, and E. J. Pellman, Concussion in Professional Football: Biomechanics of the Struck Player—Part 14. *Neurosurgery*, 2007. 61(2): 313–27; discussion 327–28.

11

THE CUMULATIVE EFFECTS OF CONCUSSION: HOW MANY IS TOO MANY?

The story of former National Football League defensive back Andre Waters has become infamous throughout the field of sports medicine. Waters played during the 1980s and 1990s for both the Philadelphia Eagles and Arizona Cardinals. Over the course of his 12-year professional career, Waters was known as a hard hitter. His reputation earned him the nickname "Dirty Waters." He sustained many concussions during his career. In fact, during an episode of HBO's *Real Sports with Bryant Gumbel*, former Harvard University football player and professional wrestler turned concussion in sports activist Christopher Nowinski described Waters's concussion history as "probably the worst concussion history that I've come across in any player."

After retirement, Waters suffered from numerous problems. He had a steady decline in his social and cognitive functioning. His memory was severely impaired. He suffered from depression. His emotions became uncontrollable. Ultimately, on November 20, 2006, several days before Thanksgiving, Andre Waters took his own life by a self-inflicted gunshot to the head.

His brain was sent to Pennsylvania pathologist Dr. Bennet Omalu. Although Waters was only 44 years old at the time of his suicide, his brain had many similarities with that of older men. In fact, some of the medical findings discovered in Waters's brain were similar to those seen in patients suffering from Alzheimer's disease. After examining several similar cases, Dr. Omalu and others concluded that multiple concussions or head traumas sustained during these individuals' football careers led to their later life problems and the findings in the brains at autopsy.

In this chapter, we will review the studies suggesting cumulative effects of multiple concussions. The interpretation of the data will be discussed.

The limitations of the data, given the recent changes in management of this injury, will also be discussed. Some guidance in determining when an athlete ought to consider retiring from collision or contact sports will be offered. A discussion of chronic traumatic encephalopathy, a more recent diagnosis made in several former NFL players, will be reviewed.

In the Sports Concussion Clinic in the Division of Sports Medicine of Children's Hospital Boston, athletes and their families often want to know whether or not it is safe to return to sports after a concussion. "How many is too many?" they often ask. This is a difficult question to answer. Only a few medical studies have investigated this question. The results are difficult to interpret, because the way in which we diagnose concussion and manage athletes who sustain concussions has changed substantially over the last 10 to 20 years. However, this chapter will discuss some of the ways in which this question can be answered.

Many clinicians will say that if an athlete has sustained three or more concussions over the course of his or her lifetime, then he or she should be removed from contact and collision sports. Although, I disagree with this practice, it is not entirely unreasonable. It is based on some medical evidence. Several studies have asked former athletes whether or not they ever sustained a sport-related concussion. Those who answered yes were asked how many they had sustained over the course of their lifetime. Then, measurements were taken of their brain function. Their memory was tested. Their reaction time was measured. The speed with which they are able to work through problems was measured. These studies showed that those athletes who reported they sustained three or more concussions during their lifetime performed worse on the tests of brain function than those athletes who reported never sustaining a concussion. They suffered more symptoms and had more subjective memory problems than those who reported fewer concussions. For this reason, many medical professionals feel that after three concussions athletes should retire from contact and collision sports, since these sports carry the highest risk of concussion.

Indeed, this will seem like a very reasonable recommendation to most readers. But before reaching such a conclusion, let us consider some aspects of these studies. Most of the former athletes questioned played sports in the 1960s through the 1980s. Those readers who were also playing sports at that time will recall that the diagnosis and management of concussions was much different at that time. In order to be diagnosed with a concussion back then, an athlete had to be knocked unconscious for so long that the game had to stop and the athletic trainer had to come onto the field and tend to the athlete.

Nowadays we know that 90 percent of concussions in sports do not involve a loss of consciousness. We know that athletes who sustain a rapid acceleration of the head followed by confusion, disorientation, nausea, headaches, imbalance, dizziness, and slowed speech have sustained a concussion. Decades ago, such athletes were not routinely diagnosed with a concussion. They were simply told they "got their bell rung," were "shaken up on the play," "got a ding," or that they "got a dinger." Therefore, I suspect that many of the athletes in those studies who reported having three or more concussions may have sustained many more concussions by today's standards.

Similarly, the management of concussion has changed considerably. During the 1960s through the 1980s, athletes who sustained a sport-related concussion were often returned to play while still suffering from the symptoms of their concussion, many on the same day of their injury. In fact, most were returned to the game only a few plays later. Missing a game or practice after a concussion was uncommon. Therefore, the poorer brain function, or "cognitive dysfunction," noted in these studies may not reflect the total number of injuries athletes sustained but, rather, the fact that they sustained multiple injuries before they were fully recovered from previous injuries. Nowadays, we no longer return athletes to play while they are still experiencing symptoms from a concussion.

As noted, medicine has not yet figured out how many concussions is too many. And in fact, it is likely no such number exists. The number of concussions that leads to permanent deficits in memory, concentration, and other cognitive processes is likely to be different for each athlete. The number that increases the risk of dementia and other problems later in life is also likely different for each person. It might depend on the timing of the concussions with respect to one another. It might depend on the genetic makeup of the athlete. It might depend on the amount of force involved with each injury. And there may be many other factors involved that no one has yet considered. As we shall see, the overall number of concussions an athlete has sustained still plays a role in decision making about whether or not the athlete should return to contact or collision sports. But it is not the only factor, or even the main factor, in making such a decision. And there is no magic number after which physicians caring for athletes mandate retirement. For some athletes, the recommendation to retire from collision or contact sports might be made after only one or two concussions. Other athletes might be cleared to return to play after six or seven.

So if there is no magic number, how can you decide when an athlete has sustained too many concussions and should consider retiring from contact or and collision sports?

Several other factors besides the overall number help make this decision. Many of these are the same factors discussed above when deciding when it is safe to return an athlete to play after a sport-related concussion. For completeness' sake, they will be reviewed here.

Force: For some athletes, as the number of concussions sustained increases, the force required to produce a concussion seems to decrease. For example, many athletes will report that their first concussion was sustained by a high force mechanism, such as a motor vehicle accident or a major blow delivered directly to the head by a larger opponent. Their second concussion was sustained by a more moderate force, such as a blow during a body check in ice hockey that witnesses recall as being a "big hit." But after the first several concussions, many athletes report developing symptoms after an accidental blow to the head by the arm of an opponent or friend. This is a concerning sign, and will prompt clinicians to discuss retirement form contact or collision sports with the athlete.

Slower recovery: Most athletes will recover from their concussions quickly, in a matter of days to weeks. As noted, in college aged athletes 90 percent of would-be completely symptom-free within 10 days of their injury. In high school aged athletes, nearly 85 percent will be symptom-free within one week of their injury. For some athletes, however, the recovery is markedly longer, lasting weeks to months. For others, they recover from their first few, concussions quickly, just as most athletes do. But as they sustain more concussions, the recovery time increases, lasting weeks to months, or in some rare cases, longer than a year. This is another concerning sign that will prompt many physicians to discuss retiring from contact or collision sports with the athlete.

Pronounced cognitive losses: As discussed previously, cognitive function refers to one's ability to think, remember, concentrate, and reason. After a concussion, many athletes lose some of their cognitive function. As they recover, they regain their cognitive abilities. Full reattainment of cognitive function is one of the requirements for returning to play. For some athletes the cognitive losses they experience at the time of injury increase as the number of concussions increases. That means, their memory, reaction time, and the speed with which they process information becomes markedly worse after, say, their fourth concussion than it was after their first. This is another concerning sign that often prompts physicians to recommend retirement.

Similarly, some athletes will regain their cognitive function very quickly after first one or two concussions. However, as the overall number of concussions they sustain throughout their lifetime increases, the amount of time required for them to regain their cognitive function after injury also increases. When this occurs, many physicians will raise the issue of retiring from contact or collision sports with the athlete.

The decision to retire an athlete from contact or collision sports is a complicated one. For most athletes, retiring from these sports has a major impact on their lives. For professional athletes, their means for earning a living is taken away. For amateur athletes and college athletes trying to make the professional leagues, they have to give up their dream of playing in the pros. They have to choose another career. For college athletes without professional aspirations, high school athletes, and younger athletes, much social activity, self-identity, and enjoyment comes from participation in contact or collision sports. These athletes' physical health is improved by participation in sports. Many clinicians, parents, teachers, and other adults underestimate the importance of sports participation in young people's lives. Often, when athletes stop playing contact and collision sports, they lose their friends. This is usually unintentional. But most of the contact these athletes have with their friends is before practice, while dressing for sports, stretching, warming up, after practice while changing and showering, and on the bus ride to games. If concussed athletes are not around during these times, they miss out on conversations, jokes, the latest gossip, and the discussions that make people friends. This can be quite devastating.

In the Sports Concussion Clinic of the Division of Sports Medicine at Children's Hospital Boston, the decision is most often made jointly, after a long discussion between the athlete, the athlete's family, other people important to the athlete, and the doctor. Often, the conversation involves a neuropsychologist, nurse practitioner, and other members of the care team. This conversation takes place over a series of visits and lasts weeks to months. It is usually initiated after one of the above findings has been noted: 1) less force seems to be required to produce a concussion; 2) the athlete appears to take longer to recover from successive concussions; 3) the athlete has more prolonged cognitive deficits after concussions than previously; or 4) the athlete has sustained many concussions. If none of these factors applies, the athlete or, for younger athletes, the athlete's parents will often initiate the conversation by asking, "How many concussions is too many?"

I tell the athlete and others involved:

1. There is some risk of long-term problems after multiple concussions.
2. No one knows how many is too many.
3. The number is likely different for each athlete.
4. We will monitor the athlete for the factors noted above, and if they occur, we need to discuss possible retirement.
5. Athletes must understand that, even without the factors discussed above, there remains some risk.
6. They must decide for themselves whether or not they are willing to take that risk.

For athletes who earn their living by playing professional sports, most will accept a certain amount of risk and will continue to play after several concussions. For those young athletes who do not seek to play professional sports, or who do not have a realistic chance of playing professional sports, most will assume less risk, and will retire from high-risk sports after fewer concussions.

Ultimately athletes make the decision to retire themselves. On rare occasions, when the risk of returning seems too great, clinicians will refuse to allow an athlete to return against his or her wishes. But this is rare. In fact, of the more than 1,000 athletes we have cared for in the Sports Concussion Clinic, I can think of only one or two cases where an athlete was forced to retire from collision or contact sports against his or her wishes as a result of concussions. And even in these cases, they were encouraged to seek a second opinion.

What are all the news stories I see regarding professional athletes and concussion about?

Recently, there has been a flurry of media activity surrounding retired professional football players who have suffered dementia and other problems years after retirement. It is suspected that many of these problems resulted from their years in football, either as a result of sustaining multiple concussions, or as a result of sustaining multiple blows to the head that did not result in concussions.

As noted, for a long time, people have suspected that multiple blows to the head might be bad for brain function. Indeed, many readers will recall statements about certain athletes in the past, meant as a joke, such as "that guy took one too many knocks to the head." While often said in jest, these types of statements, as with most jokes, had some element of truth to them.

Some physicians have also suspected that multiple blows to the head could cause problems. Dr. Martland's aforementioned article in the *Journal of the American Medical Association* in 1928 discusses a condition in boxers which he termed "punch drunk." Later, this same entity came to be known by the more medical-sounding term, *dementia pugilistica*. Boxers suffering from dementia pugilistica had difficulties with memory, thinking, and concentration. They walked abnormally with a distinct dragging of the foot or leg. They often spoke slowly, and had notable changes in their faces.

The retired football players currently being discussed in the media suffer from a very similar and perhaps identical entity, known as chronic traumatic encephalopathy.

In 2005, in the medical journal *Neurosurgery,* Bennet Omalu, the pathologist who would later describe the case of defensive back Andre Waters, described the case of a retired National Football League Player who exhibited much of the same findings as boxers suffering from dementia pugilistica. After death, this former football player underwent an autopsy. His brain was notably different from that of a normal, healthy person. As he had no known trauma or blows to the brain except for those which he experienced while playing football, these changes in the brain were attributed to injuries he had sustained while playing football. Since that time many other cases have been described by Dr. Omalu and others. Here in Boston, a group known as the Center for the Study of Traumatic Encephalopathy studies the brain of deceased, former athletes suspected of suffering from chronic traumatic encephalopathy. They have published the results of 47 cases of this condition. They have discovered it is not exclusive to football players, or to former professional athletes.

It is not clear exactly what causes chronic traumatic encephalopathy. Certainly, it seems to be related to repeated blows to the head. Many of the athletes first noted to have CTE sustained multiple concussions over their careers. This led doctors to believe that CTE resulted from multiple concussions. However, CTE has since been discovered in athletes who were not known to have suffered many concussions. It is possible that these athletes sustained multiple concussions and simply did not tell anyone about them. But it also raises the possibility that CTE does not result from the multiple concussions, but rather, from the hundreds or thousands of blows to the head that boxers and football players routinely sustain that do not cause a concussion. During nearly every play, the head of a lineman playing American football collides with his opponent. Most of these blows do not cause a concussion. But perhaps they result in some small amount of injury to the brain that, when repeated thousands of times over the course of a career, ultimately leads to chronic traumatic encephalopathy. Similarly, boxers sustain many punches to the head over their careers. Most of these punches do not result in a concussion. But perhaps each punch, even when it does not cause a concussion, results in some small amount of injury to the brain that, when repeated thousands of times over the course of a boxer's career, leads to chronic traumatic encephalopathy.

Of course, there may be other factors involved. There are many football players and boxers who do not develop the clinical signs and symptoms of CTE, even after years of play. We do not yet know what the difference is between those who develop chronic traumatic encephalopathy clinically and those who do not. Some studies have suggested that it may be due to genetic factors; some athletes may be predisposed to developing CTE after injury when compared to others. It may be due to environmental factors. Athletes taking certain medications, nutritional supplements, ergogenic aids, or vitamins may be at higher risk of CTE than others. It may have to do with the timing of the injuries. Perhaps sustaining repeated blows to the head at a certain age results in chronic traumatic encephalopathy, whereas at other ages it does not. Or it might not be related to any of these factors. Researchers are actively trying to determine which factors place athletes at risk for CTE so that we can better prevent and manage this disease.

In summary, for some athletes, multiple concussions will lead to a loss of some cognitive function that is not recovered. Some athletes who sustain multiple concussions over the course of their athletic careers will have problems later in life, including decreased cognitive abilities, dementia, mood disorders, headaches, and insomnia. The number of concussions that ultimately leads to long-term problems is unknown, and likely differs between athletes. It is likely that some athletes will sustain multiple concussions and not have long-term problems. Still others may sustain long-term problems after only a few sport-related concussions. Currently, there is no way for clinicians to tell which athletes are at risk for suffering problems later in life. There are likely multiple factors involved, including the number of injuries, the amount of force with each injury, and some underlying predisposition for long-term problems after a concussion in certain athletes. Until more is known, athletes should consider their own personal risk, the importance of high-risk sports in their lives, and their long-term career goals when making decisions to return to contact sports, collision sports, or other high-risk activities.

SUGGESTED READINGS

Cantu, R. C., Chronic Traumatic Encephalopathy in the National Football League. *Neurosurgery,* 2007. 61(2): 23–25.

Guskiewicz, K. M., et al., Association between Recurrent Concussion and Late-Life Cognitive Impairment in Retired Professional Football Players. *Neurosurgery,* 2005. 57 (4): 719–26; discussion 719–26.

Guskiewicz, K. M., et al., Cumulative Effects Associated with Recurrent Concussion in Collegiate Football Players: The NCAA Concussion Study. *JAMA,* 2003. 290(19): 2549–55.

Guskiewicz, K. M., et al., Recurrent Concussion and Risk of Depression in Retired Profes-
    sional Football Players. *Med Sci Sports Exerc*, 2007. 39(6): 903–9.
McKee, A. C., et al., Chronic Traumatic Encephalopathy in Athletes: Progressive Tauopathy
    after Repetitive Head Injury. *J Neuropathol Exp Neurol*, 2009. 68(7): 709–35.
Meehan, W. P., 3rd, P. d'Hemecourt, and R. D. Comstock, High School Concussions in the
    2008–2009 Academic Year: Mechanism, Symptoms, and Management. *Am J
    Sports Med*, 2010. 38(12): 2405–9.
Omalu, B. I., et al., Chronic Traumatic Encephalopathy in a National Football League
    Player. *Neurosurgery*, 2005. 57(1): 128–34; discussion 128–34.
Omalu, B. I., et al., Chronic Traumatic Encephalopathy in a National Football League
    Player: Part II. *Neurosurgery*, 2006. 59(5): 1086–92; discussion 1092–93.

12

THE FEMALE ATHLETE: ARE GIRLS AND BOYS DIFFERENT WHEN IT COMES TO CONCUSSION?

In January 2010, Australian snowboarder Torah Bright was considered a favorite to win the Olympic gold medal. With an inspiring performance in the 2006 Olympics, and countless other demonstrations of her ability since, Bright was favored over her two American opponents. Approximately two weeks before her bid for the Olympic gold, she was at the Winter X Games in Aspen, Colorado. During a routine training run, Bright accelerated up the side of the half pipe wall. Once airborne she completed a 540-degree turn, something she had done many times before without difficulty. This time, however, she lost control in the air. She cascaded down the wall. Her arms, rotating backward in an effort to help her regain her balance, were not in position to break her fall. The edge of her board landed first, catching on the down slope of the half pipe, and sending her body spinning. Her head snapped backward as her body landed, the back of it, striking the ground sharply. She brought her hands to her head almost immediately. She moved little until medical help arrived. With a shot at the Olympic gold medal only weeks away, she lay on the cold snow, stunned and nearly motionless.

Torah Bright was concussed.

While sport-related concussion is most commonly discussed as an injury to male athletes, it is a growing concern in the female athlete as well. It is likely that the focus on male athletes stems from their involvement in contact and collision sports. Historically, male athletes have played these sports in much greater numbers than female athletes. In the past, male athletes played much more aggressively than female athletes did. But this has changed decidedly over the last several decades. More and more female athletes are participating in contact and even collision sports, such as rugby.

Currently, over 178,000 women participate in sports sponsored by the National Collegiate Athletic Association. It is estimated that 3 million female athletes participate in high school sports. The number of women participating in contact sports, collision sports, and even combat sports is on the rise. The last several decades has seen the formation of women's leagues for collision sports such as American football and rugby as well as combat sports such as boxing. Laila Ali, the daughter of former heavyweight champion Muhammad Ali, became famous in the last decade after becoming a professional boxer. Indeed, while I was attending Boston College in the 1990s, the women's rugby team won the national championship. Along with this increase in popularity has come more aggressive and even ferocious play in women's sports. This has led to increased recognition of concussive brain injury in female athletes.

Still there are some differences between male and female athletes with respect to concussion. In terms of the percentage of female athletes sustaining a concussion within a given sport, some medical evidence suggests that female athletes are at higher risk than their male counterparts. Some medical studies conducted in sports played by both female and male athletes suggest that women suffer higher rates of concussion. Multiple investigators have noted higher rates of concussion in women's soccer and basketball than in men's soccer and basketball, both at the high school and college levels.

Several possible reasons for this discrepancy exist. Some researchers believe that female athletes are simply more honest than male athletes, reporting their injury more frequently. Others argue that perhaps the difference is cultural. Male athletes are often taught that they should "tough it out" through an injury and report that nothing bothers them even when they are injured. Several medical studies have shown that female athletes report more symptoms after sustaining sport-related concussions than male athletes. Furthermore, they tend to rank their symptoms as more severe. They often complain of having symptoms for longer periods of time than their male counterparts. Some argue that these studies provide evidence of female athletes being more honest than male athletes. However, it is equally possible that female athletes have worse symptoms and take longer to recover than male athletes. Men may be just as honest but are truly recovering more quickly. Thus far, no one has been able to tease out these two possibilities.

If it is true that women and girls are more likely to sustain concussions and to require longer recovery times than male athletes, it begs the question: why? There are several possible reasons why female athletes may be more likely to sustain concussions and may take longer to recover from concussions.

Some researchers argue that the difference is biological. As we have already learned earlier in this book, concussion is due to a rapid, rotational acceleration of the brain at the time of impact. We have also learned that by strengthening the neck muscles, athletes might reduce their risk of sustaining sport-related concussions. A medical study by athletic trainer Ryan Tierney and colleagues showed that female athletes have 49 percent less muscle strength and

30 percent less muscle girth than male athletes. Given their larger mass, larger muscle mass, and increased neck muscle strength, male athletes may be less likely to sustain sport-related concussions than female athletes competing in the same sport.

Some doctors and scientists have suggested that the different concentrations of hormones circulating in the blood may change the risks of sustaining a concussion and recovering from a concussion. In particular, it has been suggested that the female sex hormone, estrogen, may make females more susceptible to concussive brain injury. However, the exact role of estrogen is controversial. In laboratory experiments using rodents, giving estrogen to male mice has improved their outcome after a traumatic brain injury. Female rodents given extra estrogen prior to traumatic brain injuries, however, did markedly worse. Thus, the true effect of estrogen, if any, on outcome after traumatic brain injury remains unclear. Whether or not estrogen has any effect on the risk of sustaining a sport-related concussion or the recovery after suffering a sport-related concussion is unknown.

One of the advantages of computerized neuropsychological testing is that it allows us to measure or quantify the degree of injury, or brain dysfunction, after a concussion. Studies have revealed differences in cognitive function between male and female athletes. These differences are true both before and after injury. Clearly there are some differences between male and female athletes in the way the brain operates. In one study, collegiate women's soccer players who sustained a concussion had slower reaction times than male collegiate soccer players who sustained a concussion. Other studies have shown differences in memory between male and female athletes. Still, the role that these potential differences in cognitive function has on risk of sustaining a concussion or time required to recover from a concussion remains unknown.

In summary, there does appear to be differences in the risk of concussion between male and female athletes, with women and girls being at higher risk of sustaining injury. Similarly, there is some evidence suggesting that female athletes might take longer to recover from concussions than male athletes. The reasons for these potential discrepancies are unknown. Honesty in reporting, differences in muscle mass or strength, varying hormone levels, or discrepancies in cognitive abilities are all being considered as potential factors.

SUGGESTED READINGS

Broshek, D. K., et al., Sex Differences in Outcome Following Sports-Related Concussion. *J Neurosurg*, 2005. 102(5): 85–63.

Colvin, A. C., et al., The Role of Concussion History and Gender in Recovery from Soccer-Related Concussion. *Am J Sports Med*, 2009. 37(9): 1699–704.

Covassin, T., et al., Sex Differences in Baseline Neuropsychological Function and Concussion Symptoms of Collegiate Athletes. *Br J Sports Med*, 2006. 40(11): 923–27; discussion 927.

Covassin, T., C. B. Swanik, and M. L. Sachs, Sex Differences and the Incidence of
Concussions Among Collegiate Athletes. *J Athl Train*, 2003. 38(3): 238–44.

Covassin, T., P. Schatz, and C. B. Swanik, Sex Differences in Neuropsychological Function
and Post-Concussion Symptoms of Concussed Collegiate Athletes. *Neurosurgery*,
2007. 61(2): 345–50; discussion 350–51.

Farace, E., and W. M. Alves, Do Women Fare Worse? A Metaanalysis of Gender Differences in Outcome after Traumatic Brain Injury. *Neurosurg Focus*, 2000. 8(1): 6.

Gessel, L. M., et al., Concussions among United States High School and Collegiate
Athletes. *J Athl Train*, 2007. 42(4): 495–503.

Tierney, R. T., et al., Gender Differences in Head-Neck Segment Dynamic Stabilization
During Head Acceleration. *Med Sci Sports Exerc*, 2005. 37(2): 272–79.

13

SETTING UP A CONCUSSION PROGRAM

On Friday September 25, 2009, talk show host Conan O'Brien was engaged in a mini mock triathlon against *Desperate Housewives* star Teri Hatcher. The last leg of the event consisted of a footrace. As they descended the studio stairs, Hatcher had a slight lead. They mounted the stage and dashed for the finish line. Approximately 6 feet before the finish line, O'Brien's legs slid out in front of him. He fell backwards. The back of his head struck the ground with an audible "boom." Per his own report on a later show, O'Brien had confusion for several minutes after the event. He said, "In the moment, I saw stars. But I tried to keep going." He was unable to recall the year. He was unfamiliar with his remaining duties for the show. He had significant amnesia for the events following the injury.

Conan O'Brien was concussed.

That's right. Concussion doesn't only happen during organized sports. Those of us in the field of sports medicine must be prepared to care for our athletes' injuries, regardless of where or how they occur. A comprehensive concussion program will help in that effort.

Many readers will recall that in the 1980s concussion was not considered a serious injury. It is only during that decade that medical investigators started examining the effects of concussion on brain function. Much of the medical and scientific evidence reviewed in this book is relatively new. The current approaches to assessing and managing concussive brain injury are also relatively new. Many athletic trainers, physicians, neuropsychologists, and medical professionals will be unaware of some of these findings, guidelines, and recommendations. This should not be alarming. Medical information does not come about as the result of one or two studies. Medical practice changes only as a result of many studies, investigating various aspects of a medical problem, and all pointing to a similar conclusion. Given the other injuries, illnesses, and diseases that medical professionals must manage, concussion may represent a very small proportion of an individual clinician's practice. Therefore, the first step in setting up a comprehensive concussion management program will be to identify a clinician who is knowledgeable about the assessment and management of sport-related concussions. In many communities, such an individual may not be readily available. In this case, clinicians who are interested in the assessment and management of concussive brain injuries should be encouraged to review the available medical literature and start a management program from scratch.

Ideally, a comprehensive concussion management program consists of many medical professionals from different specialties as opposed to a single clinician. Ideal programs include athletic trainers, physicians, neuropsychologists, other medical clinicians such as nurse practitioners or physician assistants, sports psychologists, and physical therapists. The roles of each of these medical professionals will be discussed in further detail below.

Once clinicians have been identified who will assess and manage the sport-related concussions of a given group of athletes, they must decide collectively which standardized assessments will be used. A standard symptom inventory should be used among all clinicians for all athletes. Likewise, a standard balance assessment should be used by all clinicians and for all athletes. The balance assessment should be measured and scored in precisely the same way by all individuals participating in the program. This will allow for consistent measurements. Similarly, a single standardized sideline concussion assessment tool should be chosen so that all clinicians are performing the same sideline assessment on every athlete. Finally, a computerized neuropsychological assessment should be chosen and a baseline assessment should be performed on every athlete.

As mentioned previously there are several different symptom inventories available. Prior to the start of the season the clinicians who will be caring for the athletes should get together and decide which symptom inventory they will use. They must decide whether, during the baseline assessment, an athlete should score any particular symptom he or she is experiencing on the day of the baseline assessment, or whether all athletes who are not currently concussed at the time of the baseline assessment should score a zero. Therefore, after injury athletes would only score those symptoms that resulted from the concussion. For readers who are looking to start a comprehensive concussion management plan but are unfamiliar with symptom inventories, the Standardized Concussion Assessment Tool version 2 is available for free online and includes an excellent symptom inventory known as the post-concussion symptoms scale. At the time of this writing, typing "SCAT 2" into the *Google* search bar and clicking on the first recommended link will take you to a free, downloadable version of the SCAT 2.

Baseline balance assessment must also be obtained for every athlete prior to the start of the season. There are several versions of the balance error scoring system available. Perhaps the easiest to use and most accessible to the reader is the modified balance error scoring system proposed as part of the Standardized Concussion Assessment Tool version 2. Again, it is available for free online.

Clinicians caring for athletes must also decide on which sideline assessment they will use. This decision should be made primarily by the clinician who will be on the side of the field, ice rink, or court, and is most likely to be present when a concussive injury occurs. For most athletic teams, this will be the athletic trainer. Again, several sideline concussion assessments are available and have been reviewed previously in this book. Some are available for free online.

Finally, the group must decide which computerized neuropsychological assessment will be used. This will depend heavily on which clinicians will be caring for the athletes. Each of the computerized neuropsychological assessments uses different testing paradigms, different ways of scoring the test, and different ways of reporting athletes' scores. The clinicians, regardless of their background, need to undertake training in the specific computerized neuropsychological assessment chosen in order to correctly administer and interpret these tests. There are several versions available. Readers who are starting a comprehensive concussion management program in the area should contact a local physician or neuropsychologist experienced in the assessment and management of sport-related concussions in order to determine which computerized neuropsychological assessment will be best for their program. If no such clinician is available in your area, athletic trainers can often be useful in identifying a doctor or other clinician who might be interested in collaborating in a comprehensive concussion management program.

In most cases, the athletic trainer will coordinate the baseline assessments of the athletes, ensuring that a baseline symptom inventory, a baseline balance assessment, a baseline sideline assessment, and a baseline computerized neuropsychological test is obtained for every athlete. As the athletic trainer will often be on the sidelines, courtside, or rink side when concussive injury occurs, it is the athletic trainer who will be responsible for repeating the sideline assessment when diagnosing an athlete with a sport-related concussion. The athletic trainer will ensure that the athlete is not returned to sport until completely recovered from the concussion. The athletic trainer will coordinate all required follow-up and medical appointments.

The team physician's presence can vary based on availability, team resources, and other factors. Ideally the team physician is present at all competitions. For many teams, the athletic trainer will respond first to all injuries. The team physician will be available to the athletic trainer for any injury that should require further medical assessment. In other settings, the athletic trainer and team physician will respond to injury simultaneously. In some circumstances, the team physician may not be present at competitions. In these situations the team physician's role is to see the athletes in clinic, provide further assessment, treatment, and coordinate all outpatient care. In an ideal program, the athletic trainer and team physician work closely together.

Nurse practitioners and physician assistants function similarly to the team physician, and usually under the guidance or supervision of the team physician. While in some cases they may be present at athletic events, their main role is in the clinic, where they will assess and manage injuries on an out-patient basis.

Many teams may have a designated neuropsychologist who works closely with the team physician in the assessment and management of sport-related concussions. Neuropsychologists will help make the diagnosis of the sport-related concussion, particularly in situations where the diagnosis may be somewhat unclear. They may administer and interpret both computerized neuropsychological tests as well as traditional neuropsychological tests in order to ascertain an athlete's brain function. They will prescribe therapies and strategies to help an athlete recover from his or her concussion. They will provide academic accommodations for student athletes, which allow athletes to safely participate in school while recovering from their concussions. They will help determine when an athlete has recovered from his or her concussion. They will guide the athlete in safely returning to play.

As noted previously, while most athletes will have recovered from their concussions relatively quickly, a minority of athletes will take several weeks to months to recover completely from their sport-related concussions. Such prolonged recoveries can often have negative effects on an athlete's mood, behavior, and overall disposition. In these circumstances, a sports psychologist, or, if a sports psychologist is unavailable, a general psychologist, will be useful in counseling, teaching coping strategies, and assessing for more serious mood disorders. While few teams will have a dedicated sports psychologist, most team physicians will have a sports psychologist with whom they work closely and may refer athletes in need.

The physical therapist in most concussion programs will be used to prepare an athlete who sustains a sport-related concussion for a safe return to sports. As noted previously, once the athlete is recovered he or she should not be returned directly into competition, especially after a period of prolonged rest. After long periods of rests, athletes become weaker, slower. They lose some of their agility and confidence. Their strength, conditioning, speed, reaction time, and confidence, all need to be restored prior to returning to competition. Therefore, athletes who have recently recovered from a concussion will start by engaging in some light aerobic activity. They will advance along several return-to-play stages in a stepwise fashion, advancing to more rigorous forms of exercise only if they remain symptom-free at previous levels. Physical therapists can help monitor this return to play. They can ensure that prior to returning to competition an athlete is fast, agile, strong. Returning to play prior to achieving adequate speed, agility, and strength places an athlete at increased risk for any sport related injury, not only concussion. Therefore, these important phases of return to play should not be ignored. Standard return-to-play stages, from the Second International Conference on Concussion in Sports are shown in Table 13.1.

Table 13.1
Return-to-Play Stages.

Step	Level of activity
1	No activity, complete rest. Once asymptomatic, proceed to level 2.
2	Light aerobic exercise such as walking or stationary cycling, no resistance training
3	Sport specific exercise -for example, skating in hockey, running in soccer; progressive addition of resistance training at steps 3 or 4.
4	Non-contact training drills.
5	Full contact training after medical clearance.
6	Game play.

Once all personnel have been identified, have agreed to participate, and have been appropriately trained in assessing and managing sport-related concussions, baseline assessments should be made and the concussion management team should meet and discuss a plan of action. The plan of action should include which preseason baseline assessments will be performed, who will perform them, and when they will be performed. The plan should include guidelines for the acute response to injury, for the clinical, outpatient management, and for return to play. Below is an example of a concussion action plan. These plans of action are most effective if written down and distributed to all medical personnel, coaches, parents, and other people involved with the team.

A concussion action plan, or concussion protocol, is a written document developed by all members of the sports medicine team. It consists of seven major components.

I. The definition of concussion. The concussion action plan often starts by defining concussive brain injury and describing some of the characteristics of a concussion, including some of the ways athletes sustain concussions.
II. The signs and symptoms of concussion. Often, the concussion action plan will contain lists or tables that review for the sports medical team the signs and symptoms most often associated with sport-related concussions.
III. Preseason items. All actions that should be performed prior to the start of the season are described in this section of the concussion action plan. The baseline assessments that the sports medicine team has chosen to obtain on all at-risk athletes will be described in this section. Any cervical muscle strengthening or other preventative strategies will also be included here.
IV. On-site response to injury. This section details the immediate response to an injured athlete. It should review proper techniques for immobilizing an athlete and transporting an athlete to a local emergency department when necessary. For athletes who sustain less emergent injuries, specifics are given for monitoring

the athlete after injury. Often this section will include instructions to be given to the athlete, the athlete's roommates or family members, and others who will be with the athlete for the 24 hours following the injury.

V. Outpatient response to injury. This section describes how the athlete will be managed during the days and weeks following a sport-related concussion. It will describe which providers are involved in the care of the concussed athlete. It will describe some initial therapies as well as which members of the larger team or school community need to be notified. Concussion action plans at academic institutions will often include academic planning and how academic accommodations can be put into place for the concussed athlete. Which members of the sports medicine team will discuss the situation with school administrators is often discussed in this section. Usually, this part of the concussion action plan includes the requirements for determining when an athlete has completely recovered from his or her concussion.

VI. Off-campus injuries. Although it is most common for athletes to sustain their concussions while participating in sports, concussions also occur outside of sports. The truly detailed concussion action plan includes an approach to assessing and treating those concussions that occur outside of organized sports activity.

VII. Return to play. Specific guidelines for returning an athlete to play who has recently recovered from a sport-related concussion are discussed. The stages that must precede the return to game play, the monitoring of the stages, and the specific activities allowed during each stage are often outlined in this section.

Not all concussion action plans are the same. Not all contain every section. Others may contain information not mentioned here. The action plan should be tailored to suit the needs of the athletes covered by it. It should be adjusted to account for the circumstances, sports being played, type of sports equipment being worn, playing surfaces, number of personnel involved, type of personnel involved, and available resources. In order to give the reader an idea of what a concussion action plan looks like, one is included below. It is based on the concussion action plan developed by Rick Burr, the head athletic trainer at Babson College, in Waltham, Massachusetts. It has been adjusted slightly to be more generic and perhaps applicable to your team. Some of the terms are in medical jargon, and you may not be familiar with their meaning. However, this template can be used by the medical personnel involved in your concussion protocol, who will be familiar with these terms. In addition, several of the appendices noted in this sample concussion action plan are included elsewhere in this book, and therefore not duplicated here.

In order to illustrate how an effective concussion action plan works, two stories are included as follows. One story is of an athlete who has sustained a relatively straightforward injury. The other is of an athlete who has sustained a concussion that has resulted in a more complicated and drawn-out course. The names used are fictional. The stories themselves do not represent any specific athlete.

CONCUSSION PROTOCOL FOR YOUR TEAM

Concussion can be defined as a traumatic injury to the brain as a result of a violent blow to the head, shaking of the head, or spinning of the head.

POSSIBLE CAUSES OR MECHANISMS OF INJURY (MOI) OF A CONCUSSION

Direct or Indirect Blows

Blow to the head, face, neck, back, or jaw can all result in a concussion.

- Blow to the body, jarring impact, even if the head isn't immediately impacted. The head may be shaken or jarred violently without impacting the ground or other object.
- Significant whiplash or similar injury to the head/neck/back region.

COMMON SIGNS AND SYMPTOMS OF SPORTS-RELATED CONCUSSION

Signs (observed by medical professionals, teammates, or others):

- Athlete appears dazed or stunned
- Confusion (about instructions, plays, etc.)
- Forgets plays/cannot recall recent events
- Unsure about game details, score, opponent
- Moves clumsily (altered coordination), has balance problems
- Personality change, uncontrolled emotions (crying or angry)
- Responds slowly to questions, has to think about answers
- Forgets events prior to a hit
- Forgets events after a hit
- Loss of consciousness (any duration)

Symptoms (reported by an athlete):

- Headache, pressure in the head
- Fatigue, wants to sleep, feels sluggish
- Nausea or vomiting
- Double vision, blurry vision
- Sensitive to light, noises, or smells
- Feels dazed or stunned
- Feels "foggy"
- Problems concentrating
- Problems remembering

These signs and symptoms are indicative of probable concussion. Other causes for symptoms should also be considered.

RED FLAGS! When these occur, the athlete should be transported IMMEDIATELY via ambulance to the emergency department

- Seizure
- Loss of consciousness
- Repeated vomiting
- Dilated pupils
- Severe neck pain
- Inability to recognize faces
- Tingling/weakness in arms or legs
- Slurred speech
- Worsening headache
- Inability to stay awake
- Altered consciousness

NOTE! Any athlete who is unconscious should be treated as if he or she has a head **and neck** injury, potentially a cervical spine injury!

Baseline Testing

ImPACT Neuropsychological Testing

About ImPACT

- ImPACT (Immediate Post-Concussion Assessment and Cognitive Testing) is a research-based software tool utilized to evaluate recovery after concussion.
- ImPACT evaluates multiple aspects of neurocognitive function, including memory, attention/concentration, brain processing speed, reaction time, and post-concussion symptoms
- Neuropsychological testing is utilized to help determine recovery after concussion.

All athletes at high to moderate risk (soccer, field hockey, basketball, ice hockey, diving, alpine skiing, baseball, softball, lacrosse) are required to take a baseline ImPACT test prior to the first day of participation in that sport. Also included will be athletes with a prior history of a concussion participating in less risky sports. No athlete will be allowed to take part in the sport until ImPACT testing is complete.

GUIDELINES AND PROCEDURES FOR COACHES

Recognize, Remove, Refer!

Recognize Concussion
- All coaches should be familiar with the signs and symptoms of concussions that are described on the first page of this document.
- Athletes should be monitored for changes in mental status.

Remove from Activity
- If the coach suspects an athlete has sustained a concussion, the athlete should be removed from activity immediately, and remain out of sports until evaluated.
- If at an away competition, the host athletic trainer decisions regarding playing status are *final*.

Refer the Athlete to Be Evaluated
- If at an away competition, athletes should present signs and symptoms to the host athletic trainer.
- Coaches should report all head injuries to Babson College Sports Medicine staff on returning to campus.

GUIDELINES FOR STUDENT ATHLETES

All student athletes will be presented with a Concussion Education program as part of the NCAA Pre-Participation Seminar conducted annually prior to the first day of practice. Student athletes will also sign, as part of their Consent Agreement, a statement of recognition that it is the student athlete's responsibility to report all concussions or concussion-like symptoms to the Sports Medicine Staff within 24 hours of the onset. Student athletes also understand it is the sole responsibility of the Sports Medicine Staff to manage the return-to-play criteria following all injuries including concussions.

ON THE FIELD MANAGEMENT

Suggested Guidelines for Management of Concussions at Your School

Assessment of Cognitive Function and Coordination
General cognitive status should be determined by sideline cognitive testing performed by the Athletic Trainer on site.

- Sports Concussion Assessment Tool

Any athlete with a witnessed loss of consciousness (LOC) of **any duration** shall be transported by EMS.

Any athlete who has symptoms of a concussion, and who is not stable (i.e., condition is changing or deteriorating), should also be transported immediately via EMS.

An athlete who exhibits any of the following symptoms, or other concerning symptoms, shall be transported immediately via EMS.

- deterioration of neurological function
- decreasing level of consciousness
- decrease in or irregularity of respirations
- any irregularity in pulse
- unequal, dilated, or nonreactive pupils
- any signs or symptoms of associated injuries, spine or skull fracture, or bleeding
- mental status changes such as lethargy, difficulty maintaining arousal, confusion or agitation
- seizure activity
- any focal neurological deficit

SUGGESTED GUIDELINES FOR CONCUSSIONS THAT HAPPEN OFF CAMPUS

Athletes/coaches will follow recommendations of the host Athletic Trainer.

- If recommended by the host Athletic Trainer, athletes should be taken to the hospital closest to the site of competition for prompt evaluation.
- Sports Medicine Staff should be notified as soon as possible after these events.
- The Director of Athletics shall be notified as well as the Public Safety and Campus Life departments
- All symptoms must be reported for the purposes of developing or modifying an appropriate health care plan for the student athlete.
- The Sports Medicine staff is responsible for monitoring recovery and coordinating the appropriate return to play activity progression.

If the student athlete is allowed to return to the dorms or go home with their parents, they will be given a Head Injury sheet explaining all recommendations for the student athlete, including actions to take if symptoms become worse. The student athlete will set up a time to meet with the Sports Medicine staff the next day, when possible, to reassess the injury.

MANAGEMENT OF THE CONCUSSION

Whether evaluated on site or reported through another source, the following steps will constitute the protocol for concussion evaluation and return to any physical activity under the direct supervision of Sports Medicine Staff:

Step 1

Immediate Post-Concussion Assessment and Cognitive Testing* (ImPACT) is administered within forty-eight hours of the evaluation by an certified Athletic Trainer, unless the student athlete is unable to perform the test without causing worsening of the athlete's symptoms.

a. The results are compared to the student athlete's baseline testing for any noticeable discrepancies. If there is no baseline data for the student athlete then the athletic trainer will follow protocol and compare to national norms, provided by the ImPACT database.

b. If the results of the post injury ImPACT test are comparable to baseline, and the athlete has no symptoms, the Athletic Trainers will move forward with exertion tests for returning the athlete to play.

c. If one or more testing areas demonstrate significant or question-able decline when compared to the baseline, then the test scores will be reviewed by the designated concussion medical team. Should the cognitive scores appear reassuring (some concussions present that way) but there is a presence of post-concussive symptoms, then the concussion medical team will also assess the case. Appointments will be made to follow-up the care of the student athlete. The class Dean will be made aware of special accommodations for academic needs. It could be recommended that the student athlete avoid all stimuli, including class work, for a period of time.

d. The concussion medical team will inform the athletic trainer of specific steps to take, based on the testing results and post-concussive symptoms. If the concussion medical team recommends more testing, then Your School will adhere to the time frame given before moving to the exertion test.

Step 2

When the concussion medical team advises that the athlete is ready for physical exertion, then an Athletic Trainer will perform the following testing:

Stage 1
Under the supervision of an Athletic Trainer, the student athlete will perform 15–20 minutes of supervised light cardio exercises. Target Heart rate should be 30–40 percent of maximal exertion.

Recommended Exercises:
- Stationary bike, walking on treadmill (10–15 minutes)
- Light hand weights, or resistive band rowing
- Stretching: quads, calf, hamstring
- Single leg balance

Stage 2
Under the supervision of an Athletic Trainer, and if still symptom-free, the student athlete will perform 30–45 minutes of supervised light to moderate cardio and low level type exercises. Target Heart Rate 40–60 percent of maximal exertion.

Recommended Exercises:
- Treadmill, Stationary bike, elliptical, UBE (20–25 minutes)
- Light weight strengthening exercises, resistive band work, wall squats, lunges, step up/down
- Stage 1 stretching, active stretching as tolerated (lung walk, side to side, walking hamstring)
- Romberg's exercises, VOR exercises (walking with eyes focused with head turn). Swiss ball exercises, single leg balance

Stage 3
Under the supervision of an Athletic Trainer, and if still symptom-free, Moderately Aggressive Aerobic Exercise. 60–80 percent of maximum heart rate.

Recommended Exercises:
- Treadmill, stationary bike, elliptical, UBE (25–30 minutes)
- Resistive weight training including free weights; MRS/functional squats. Dynamic strength activities
- Active stretching
- Initiate agility drills (zigzags, side shuttle, jumping on blocks/tramp)
- Higher level balance activities: ball toss on plyo-floor, balance disc, trampoline, BOSU work

Stage 4

Under the supervision of an Athletic Trainer and if still symptom-free, Noncontact Physical Training. 80 percent of maximum heart rate.
Sport Specific activities
Conclusion retest ImPact

Stage 5

If balance and neurocognitive function have returned to baseline and the athlete is still symptom-free, the student athlete my resume full physical training activity with contact, under the supervision of a Babson College Athletic Trainer.
Resume Full Activity

If at any time symptoms return, the concussion medical team will be notified. For athletes with a history of multiple concussions, prolonged recoveries, injuries that occur with only minimal force or other concerning circumstances, the return–to–play timeline may be adjusted.

AFTERCARE INSTRUCTION SHEET

HEAD INJURY

You have suffered a head injury. Even though you are being allowed to go to your dorm or home, a relative or friend should stay with you. **You both should read the following instructions:**
During the first 24 hours:

1. Eat and drink little. Clear liquids are best if your stomach is upset.
2. Drink **NO** alcoholic beverages.
3. Relax in bed if possible. Do not exert yourself in any way.
4. Do not take sedatives or sleeping pills.
5. Do not drive a car or motorized equipment.
6. Try to nap or sleep more than usual.
7. If you have lost consciousness ("passed-out") following a head injury, we advise that you not be allowed to sleep for periods longer than two hours without being aroused. You should not be left alone.

8. Avoid aspirin, ibuprofen, or compounds containing them. Use acetaminophen (Tylenol) instead.
9. Avoid watching television, using computers, playing video games, working online, text-messaging, and reading.

If any of the following symptoms appear, go directly to the Emergency Department immediately:

1. Persistent nausea or vomiting.
2. Confusion, unusual drowsiness, or loss of memory.
3. Dizziness, trouble walking or staggering.
4. Convulsions or seizures ("fits"). These are twitching or jerking movements of either the eyes, arms, legs, or body.
5. Pupils of unequal size. The pupil is the dark center portion of the eye.
6. A severe headache or a headache that is worsening or persistent.
7. Personality changes.
8. Weakness or trouble with the use of arms or legs; or areas of skin numbness.
9. Unconsciousness or fainting.
10. Stiff neck or fever.
11. Visual disturbances including blurring of vision and double vision.
12. Unusual sounds in the ear(s), such as ringing.
13. Bleeding or clear liquid drainage from the ears or nose.
14. Difficulty speaking or slurred speech.
15. Excessive sleepiness or difficulty rousing from sleep.
16. Developing shortness of breath or difficulty breathing.
17. Any unusual or abnormal symptoms.

It is important that you report any new or remaining problems during your follow-up appointment with Sports Medicine. It is not uncommon for you to have persistent or recurring headaches following your head injury. However, those who have remaining difficulties should be followed either by their physician or Health Services. Should you have any questions or difficulties, do not hesitate to contact your own physician or go to the Emergency Department.

Brian is a 22-year-old college ice hockey player at a highly competitive New England college hockey program. Since high school, he has been actively pursued by many National Hockey League teams. He plans to play professional ice hockey after graduation. Brian's team is second in the league, and hoping to qualify for the NCAA tournament. Only two weeks remain in the season.

The score is 3 to 2. Brian's team is down by one. There are nine minutes remaining in the second period of play. Brian has the puck. He loses control of the puck as he crosses center ice. He looks down, in an attempt to regain control of the puck. He is struck in the shoulder by an opposing defensemen. He is lifted off the ice and hurled backward. As he lands, the back of his head strikes the ice sharply and bounces up. He is clearly having difficulty balancing, making several unsuccessful attempts to stand up, before he is able to steady himself and successfully skate toward the bench, all the while supporting his body weight with his hockey stick. He reports to the athletic trainer that he feels "a little out of it" and has "a killer headache." The athletic trainer walks Brian down the ramp into the hallway behind the bench, where it is somewhat quieter. He repeats the standardized assessment of concussion and compares Brian's current score to the score he had at the beginning of the season. Noting that Brian has scored significantly lower, the athletic trainer sends him into the medical room, where the team physician is waiting. He informs the coach that Brian has sustained a concussion, has been removed from play, and will not be available for the rest of the game.

Brian undergoes monitoring with repeat neurological assessments performed by the team physician every 10 to 20 minutes. Over the course of this monitoring, Brian starts to feel better, although he still has some dizziness and a headache. Approximately 2 1/2 hours after the initial injury, Brian is feeling back to normal, with the exception of a mild headache. He has been told by the team physician that he sustained a concussion. Brian and his roommate are given information about sport-related concussions. They are each given verbal and written information concerning signs and symptoms to watch for over the next day. Brian is told to avoid alcohol, to avoid exercising, and to avoid activities that require concentration, memory, and other intellectually stimulating activities. Both Brian and his roommate are instructed to seek immediate medical attention if Brian develops a worsening headache, vomiting, confusion, sleepiness such that it is difficult to awaken him, or any other concerning signs or symptoms. The team physician tells Brian to follow up in clinic in two to three days.

Over the course of the next three days Brian avoids all exercise or other forms of physical exertion. He avoids intellectually stimulating activities, including doing his homework, reading for pleasure, playing videogames, working online, and text-messaging. He sleeps as much as possible. When he follows up with the team physician three days after his injury he feels completely recovered and back to normal. He has had no headaches since the morning following his injury. He has not developed any other symptoms. The team physician clears Brian to start the return-to-play stages. He discusses this with the athletic trainer, who agrees to monitor Brian's progress.

Later that afternoon the athletic trainer observes Brian exercising on a stationary bike in their training facility. After 20 minutes of some light stationary bicycling Brian continues to feel well. He has had no headaches and no other symptoms.

He is sent home for the evening. The following day Brian returns to class and has been cleared to resume all intellectual activities, as long as they do not cause his previous symptoms to recur. That day at practice he is allowed to put on his skates. The athletic trainer takes him out onto the ice alone and allows him to skate around the rink for 15 minutes. Since Brian continues to feel well, the athletic trainer gives him a hockey stick and puck and allows him to do some agility training and puck handling drills. Since he has no recurrence of his symptoms, he is allowed to do some sprinting on his skates. He continues to feel well and is sent to the training room where he is allowed to do resistance training, weight-lifting, with the rest of the team.

The following day Brian reports that he continues to feel well, without any symptoms from his previous concussion. He has not had any headaches or other symptoms of concussion despite being allowed to lift weights with the rest of the team. Therefore, he is allowed to practice with the team. Since this is his first day back to official practice, Brian is not allowed to participate in contact training drills. He is required to wear an orange pinney. This orange pinney signifies to the coaching staff, strength and conditioning coaches, athletic trainer, team physician, and Brian's teammates that he is on restrictions and is not allowed to participate in any contact drills. Every member of the team knows that they are not allowed to bodycheck Brian and he is not allowed to bodycheck them. Brian feels well during practice. He has no further symptoms that evening.

Two days later Brian has a follow-up appointment with the team physician. In reviewing the medical records the team physician notes that Brian has suffered one previous concussion during his lifetime. It occurred four years earlier. He had approximately one day worth of symptoms with that injury. There was no loss of consciousness or amnesia associated with it.

Brian reports that he has been feeling well and back to his normal self ever since the morning after his most recent concussion. He reports that he has been performing all of his schoolwork without any difficulties or any recurrence of his symptoms. Furthermore, he reports that he has been practicing fully with the team, with the exception of contact drills, and that this physical activity has not resulted in any recurrence of his concussion symptoms.

The team physician has Brian complete a symptom inventory, as he did prior to the start of the season. Similarly, he performs a modified balance error system score as was done prior to the start of the season. He notes that Brian is completely symptom-free, scoring a zero for all symptoms on the symptom inventory. He notes that Brian's balance is steady and his balance error system score is equal to what it was prior to the start of the season. He has Brian sit down at a computer and take a computerized neuropsychological assessment, similar to the one he took prior to the beginning of the season. Brian's scores are compared to his preseason baseline scores. They reveal that his memory, reaction time, and the speed it takes him to work through problems are no different than they were prior to the start of the season. His symptoms have completely resolved. They have not returned despite full cognitive exertion and full physical exertion, although he has not participated in contact drills. The team physician therefore determines that Brian is likely recovered from his concussion. He clears him to participate in full practice. He discusses this with the athletic trainer. Brian completes his first full practice including contact. He remains symptom-free after practice. He is cleared to compete in the next game without restrictions.

In the case above, the course of Brian's concussion is fairly typical. His symptoms resolved relatively quickly. In fact, in his case, they resolved in less than 24 hours. Medical studies conducted on college athletes show that approximately 90 percent will have full resolution of their concussion symptoms within 10 days of injury. Medical studies conducted in high school aged athletes reveal that nearly 85 percent will have full resolution of their symptoms and be considered recovered by their athletic trainers within seven days of their injury, 98.5 percent within one month of their injury. However, for a small percentage of athletes, their sport-related concussions can be far more troublesome. The case below describes a more complicated course that is experienced by this unfortunate minority.

Sally is a 14-year-old high school freshman. Described by her teachers as intelligent, motivated, and energetic, Sally is truly the epitome of the all-American girl. Her midterm grades were remarkable, with three As, two A minuses, and one B plus. This is all the more impressive considering that four of her classes are honors classes. She is on the yearbook committee. She is captain of her freshman soccer team. She is planning on swimming varsity in the winter and trying out for the track team in the spring.

The Wednesday before Thanksgiving Sally is playing in a freshman soccer game against one of the other local schools. She is playing left wing when a corner kick from one of her teammates drifts across the net towards the goal post nearest her. She charges forward. The right fullback for the opposing team and the opposing goalie also make a play for the ball. Out of the corner of her eye Sally sees the opposing goalie leave the net and sprint towards her. She leaps upward intending to head the ball and knock it into the upper right hand corner of the goal, past the onrushing goal keeper. However, the goal tender makes one last lunge for the ball, leading with both fists and her right knee. The two collide. The goalie's left hand punches the ball, clearing it from the goalie box. The goalie's right hand strikes Sally in the jaw. Sally falls backward, colliding with the right fullback, who is also making a play for the ball. As she falls to the ground, the back of Sally's head strikes the turf and bounces forward. The referee blows the whistle and charges the goalie with unsportsmanlike conduct. Sally's teammates notice that she is slow to rise. As they move toward her it becomes clear that she is unconscious. They wave the coach onto the field. The coach calls for the athletic trainer. Since the school only has one athletic trainer, one of the players from the bench must run over to the football field where the athletic trainer is caring for the athletes playing boys' football.

On hearing that someone has been knocked unconscious, the athletic trainer grabs her rescue bag and sprints toward the girls soccer field. On her arrival, Sally is awake but clearly confused. Her coach and fellow teammates report that Sally was unconscious for approximately 45 seconds. Since awakening she has been asking multiple times why she is on the ground. Despite being told that she was knocked down during a collision with the other team's goalie, Sally continues to ask why she is lying on the ground. The athletic trainer instructs Sally not to move. She places a hard plastic collar around Sally's neck, which prevents her neck from moving. She sends one of the other soccer players into the school to call for an ambulance. She shines a light into Sally's eyes, and asks her a series of questions. Sally does not respond to the athletic trainers questions, but rather she continuously asks why she is on the ground. Approximately six minutes later an ambulance arrives. Sally is taken to a local emergency room.

When she arrives at the emergency department Sally continues to ask why she is lying on the ground. She vomits. Given her confusion, the new onset of vomiting, and the way she appears to the doctors who examine her, Sally is taken down the hall to get a picture of her brain known as a computed tomogram or "CT scan." She has an intravenous line, or "IV," placed into her left arm. She is given a medication to help her feel less nauseous and some intravenous fluids through her IV. Just then her parents arrive. They are told by the emergency department physician that Sally has sustained a concussion. They are told that the CT scan of her brain showed that there was no swelling of the brain, no bleeding of the brain, and no skull fracture. They suspect that she will recover fully, but since she remains confused and is vomiting, they would like to observe her in the emergency department for several hours.

Over the next few hours, while in the emergency department, Sally starts to return to normal. She stops asking the same questions over and over again. She realizes that she is no longer on the field lying on the ground but rather in a hospital emergency department. She is no longer vomiting. She recognizes her parents as well as the emergency department doctor. She starts complaining of a headache. She seems slow to respond to questions and at times is somewhat disoriented, unable to answer what day of the week it is or how she arrived in the emergency department. She is able to recall taking a Spanish quiz earlier that afternoon. She is able to remember the start of the soccer match. But she cannot recall the name of the team against whom she was playing, nor what the score was. She does not remember being injured. She does not remember her journey to the hospital. She is given some crackers and ginger ale, which she is able to eat without vomiting. The emergency department physician tells her she should stay out of sports for one week. Her parents are allowed to take her home.

Throughout Thanksgiving Day and the weekend that follows, Sally continues to have headaches. She is nauseous off and on throughout the day. She notices while doing her homework that she has difficulty concentrating, often reading the same sentence multiple times over but still unable to recall its contents. She has trouble with her memory, which she notes while studying for an upcoming quiz in American history. She lies awake at night unable to sleep. At times, she feels unsteady on her feet, particularly while going up or down stairs. Her mother has been giving her acetaminophen and ibuprofen to help treat her headaches. Neither of these medications has a significant effect. When she is nauseous, Sally has been drinking ginger ale. Again this seems to have little effect.

Sally returns to school on Monday. She notices that by the end of the school day her headaches have become much worse. She is extremely nauseous and unable to eat. Over the course of the next few days, she notices that she feels somewhat better in the morning. But her headaches, nausea, and other symptoms seem to get worse as the day progresses. Ultimately she returns to soccer practice but finds that running, dribbling the ball, and other drills seem to make her headaches and other symptoms worse. She reports to the athletic trainer, who is surprised to hear that she was playing soccer again so soon. The athletic trainer removes her from practice and instructs Sally to avoid exercise until she is feeling completely back to normal. Furthermore, she recommends that Sally follow up with her pediatrician.

When Sally's mother hears this, she immediately calls the pediatrician's office and schedules a follow-up appointment. Sally sees her pediatrician the following week. Her pediatrician informs Sally's mother that the emergency department physician was mistaken. Sally should remain out of sports "for one week after her symptoms resolve, not one week after the injury occurred." Otherwise, she reports, Sally is well and should recover shortly.

As the weeks go on, however, Sally realizes that her symptoms are not gone. While her headaches may not be as intense as they were during the first few days after injury, and may not be occurring as frequently as they were during the first few days after injury, she is still having headaches by the end of almost every day. She finds herself nauseous on nearly a daily basis. Her academic performance has suffered. Her grades have gone from mostly As to mostly Cs and Ds on nearly all of the homework assignments, quizzes, and tests since her injury. She has lost touch with many of her friends with whom she used to play soccer. Since she is no longer at practice, around in the locker room, on the bus rides to away games, and other times when her friends hang out, she misses out on all of the fun, jokes, stories, and discussions that occur during these times. She finds herself exhausted at the end of the day, having much less energy throughout the day than she had prior to her injury. She has stopped many of the extracurricular activities in which she used to be involved. Her mother notices she has become quite irritable and, at times, seems frankly depressed. She has been taking acetaminophen and ibuprofen multiple times per day and still is having persistent headaches. She has gained some weight, which both Sally and her mother attribute to the fact that she is not exercising. Her mother becomes concerned by all of this and schedules another appointment with her pediatrician.

The following week Sally again sees her pediatrician. The pediatrician performs a very thorough examination. She shines a light into Sally's eyes and it uses a special scope to look into Sally's eyes. She tests Sally's reflexes. She tests Sally's balance with her eyes open and closed. She has Sally perform various tests of coordination. She tests Sally's strength throughout her muscles. In the end, the pediatrician informs both Sally and her mother that her examination is normal. She reminds them that the CT scan of Sally's brain is normal. She suggests that perhaps there is a psychological component to Sally's symptoms and offers to send her to counseling. However, both Sally and her mother are convinced that her current symptoms have resulted from her concussion. Later that evening, Sally's mother conducts an online computer search and finds a local physician who specializes in the assessment and management of sport-related concussions. She makes Sally an appointment for the following week.

On hearing of Sally's injury, the sports concussion specialist asks whether or not Sally had any balance measurements, symptom inventories, or computerized neuropsychological testing performed prior to the start of the season, or at any other time prior to her injury. Both Sally and her mother report that she had not undergone any preseason assessments. In fact, they have never heard of such a thing being done. The doctor then asks whether or not Sally has ever sustained a prior sport-related concussion or other concussion occurring outside of sports. Although never officially diagnosed with a concussion, Sally does recall falling off of her skateboard approximately five years earlier and banging her head on the sidewalk. She remembers having two to three days' worth of headaches and nausea after that incident but believes she was otherwise well. The specialist tells her that this too was a concussion. She has had two concussions over the course of her lifetime.

Sally completes a concussion symptom inventory for the specialist. Her total score on this post- concussion symptoms scale is 88. The concussion specialist then tells Sally and her mother that a concussion is a brain injury. As a result of her concussion, Sally's brain is not working properly. He believes that Sally remains symptomatic from her most recent concussion. There are several potential reasons why Sally has not yet recovered from her concussion. First of all, he knows that she has sustained a previous concussion. He informs Sally and her mother that it often takes athletes a longer time to recover from concussions when they have had other concussions previously. Second, he notes that Sally had a very small period of physical rest after her injury. Indeed, she returned to running and even practicing with the soccer team before she had completely recovered from her concussion. He explains that this sort of physical exertion prior to recovery may increase the duration of recovery and make an athlete's symptoms worse. Further, he notes that Sally has been participating fully in school. Much like exercise, cognitive exertion can also make an athlete's symptoms worse and delay recovery. Cognitive exertion, he explains, is a medical term used to describe activities that require memory, concentration, reasoning, learning, or studying. Finally, the doctor explains that by taking acetaminophen and ibuprofen every day, Sally may be making her headaches worse. While these medications are very effective when taken on occasion to treat a headache, their daily use often results in a sort of dependence that leads to what are known as rebound headaches. Rebound headaches can occur when an athlete who has been taking these medicines regularly tries to stop taking them.

Both Sally and her mother are relieved to know that she is not going crazy. They are both pleased to have an explanation for the cause of her symptoms and an explanation as to why it is taking her so much longer to recover from her concussion than they expected. At the same time, her mother has some difficulty believing that her symptoms are still due to her concussion. She has several questions.

1. How can Sally have an injury to her brain when the CT scan of her brain was normal?
2. Why did he say a concussion was an injury to the brain? She remembers her brothers being told they had concussions when they were younger. Yet they were perfectly fine, often returning to sports the very next day.
3. Why is it that they were not told any of this before?

The concussion specialist answers her questions one at a time. He explains that a CT scan is a picture of the brain. It is useful for determining whether or not a patient has sustained a structural injury to the brain. Structural injuries are things like swelling, bleeding, bruises, or cuts to the brain. A concussion, he explains, is not a structural injury. Rather, it is a functional injury. Although the brain is not bruised or swollen, it is not working properly. An athlete with a concussion will have a poor memory, slowed reaction time, and difficulty concentrating. It will take a concussed athlete longer to perform tasks that he or she used to be able to do quite easily. Since a CT scan is a picture of the brain, as opposed to a measurement of brain function, problems with brain function cannot be seen on a CT scan.

He explains further that when Sally's mother and uncles were growing up, very little was known about concussive brain injury. In fact, the term *concussion* was seldom used. Often, an athlete who sustained a concussion was described as having "had his bell rung," or having been "shaken up on the play." A concussion was thought only to have occurred when an athlete was knocked unconscious for so long that he was removed from the game and taken to a local emergency department. However, medical studies performed over the last 20 to 30 years have revealed that what used to be referred to as "bell ringers" or "dings" are actually concussions to the brain, injuries that result in measurable brain dysfunction that lasts for days to weeks after a concussive brain injury.

Finally, he informs her that much of the medical evidence regarding sport-related concussions has only been discovered in the last several years. Given the vast amount of information that a pediatrician or emergency medicine physician is required to learn, it is not surprising that she had not heard any of this previously. The recommendations for waiting a week after injury or a week after an athlete's symptoms resolved were in fact the standard medical recommendations until fairly recently. However, these recommendations were changed in light of new medical evidence.

In order to speed Sally's recovery, the sports concussion specialist recommends physical rest. This means that Sally should not exercise in any way, including jogging, swimming, bicycling, aerobic activity, push-ups, sit-ups, or any other form of exercise. Further, he recommends a period of what he terms full "cognitive rest." He explains to Sally and her mother that for the next five days, he recommends she remain home from school. He recommends she not engage in any homework, reading, video game playing, working online, text messaging, or any other activities that involve memory or concentration. This includes reading for pleasure, such as newspapers and magazines. At the end of these five days of full physical rest and full cognitive rest, he expects Sally to feel markedly better than she does currently. He does not believe she will be totally recovered by then, but rather significantly improved. At that time, she should return to school.

As her schoolwork and the activities of the school day have proven to make her symptoms worse, he recommends returning to school in stages. As opposed to taking her current seven classes, he recommends perhaps starting with three or four classes. He recommends trying to keep up in classes that build upon themselves, for example, math class. It is very difficult to learn the math that is taught in January without having first learned the math that was taught in December. Often, what is taught in January is based on what was learned in December. Math, therefore, is a class that builds upon itself. Science is a similar topic, as are languages such as Spanish or French, which tend to build on themselves. Alternatively, English literature classes tend not to build on one another. The student is able to read *Pride and Prejudice* whether or not he or she has previously read *Moby Dick*. Understanding one book does not depend on understanding the other. Therefore, even if a student missed reading one book in December, he or she is perfectly capable of reading the other book in January.

In addition he prescribes what he calls "academic accommodations." Academic accommodations, he explains, will allow Sally to have extra time on tests and quizzes. They will allow her extensions on her homework assignments. They will allow for her to take frequent breaks during the day and to go to the school nurse's office to lie down when her symptoms are troubling her. They request that she be given preprinted class notes so that she may focus on what the teacher is saying during class, as opposed to trying to write it all down for future studying. He explains to Sally and her mother that the goal of these academic accommodations is to allow Sally to keep up with her schoolwork as best as she can without making her concussion symptoms worse. Ultimately, she is responsible for making up all homework assignments, quizzes, and tests that she postpones during her recovery period. In rare circumstances, athletes have to make up missed schoolwork during the summer break.

He believes that this period of full physical and cognitive rest, followed by a period of relative cognitive rest in which Sally is allowed to return to school but is given special accommodations and some limitations on her activities, will allow her to recover from her concussion while still keeping up with the activities of her life. He asks that she return to the clinic in two or three weeks so he can see how she is doing. If she is not significantly improved at that time there are other options they might consider.

Over the five days of full physical full cognitive rest Sally starts to feel markedly improved. Her headaches become much less frequent. When she does get headaches, they are much less intense, much less painful. She is still plagued by insomnia. However, her concentration and memory seem to be improving, although she has not been engaging in activities that require a lot of concentration or memory, per her doctor's instructions. As she returns to school her symptoms increase slightly. However, she still feels better than she had prior to the five days of full rest. At her follow-up appointment with the concussion specialist, her total score on the post-concussion symptoms scale has decreased from a prior score of 88 to a current score of 29. Her main problem is headaches, which she still experiences almost daily, mostly at the end of each day. At their worst she rates them a five on a scale from zero to six, where zero is no headache whatsoever and six is the most intense, worst headache she can imagine. She is still suffering from insomnia, finding it difficult to achieve more than five hours of sleep per night. She reports to the doctor that when she is able to get six to eight hours of sleep, her headaches are often improved the following day. On returning to school she was again bothered by the difficulty she was having with her memory and concentration. Per his recommendation she is only taking four classes. However, she still finds this difficult. Her grades remain lower than usual.

The concussion specialist recommends trying an over-the-counter medication known as melatonin. Melatonin, he explains, is a hormone secreted by the brain in normal, healthy people in response to darkness. This is one of the reasons why we all become tired when it is dark outside. Melatonin, he explains, can also be purchased in a pill form. There are no significant side effects, as it is a naturally occurring hormone already circulating in her bloodstream. Getting herself some extra melatonin may help her fall asleep at night and stay asleep until morning. This, in turn, may make her headaches and other symptoms better.

He tells Sally and her mother that she is well beyond the typical duration of symptoms for a sport-related concussion despite a period of full physical and cognitive rest. Thus, he is ordering a magnetic resonance image the brain, also known as an MRI. While he suspects Sally's injury is truly a concussion and concussion alone, the MRI will rule out other possible causes of her symptoms.

In addition, he orders an electrocardiogram (EKG) of her heart in preparation for possibly offering Sally a different medical therapy at the next visit. The electrocardiogram, the doctor explains, is similar to the beeping monitors often seen on television where every time the actor's heart beats, the green line on the monitor screen develops a series of squiggles. If Sally's MRI is normal, as he expects it will be, and she has not had significant improvement in her symptoms while on the melatonin, he may offer her a medicine called amitriptyline.

In order to take amitriptyline, he explains, a person needs to have a normal heart. Although girls her age have normal hearts, he wishes to order the EKG to make sure her heart is normal, prior to prescribing amitriptyline.

Finally, he asks that Sally schedule an appointment with a neuropsychologist in the area who treats a lot of patients with concussive brain injury. Although it may take several weeks before they are able to get the appointment, he feels that this is important, as it will yield a more complete assessment of Sally's brain function. This will enable the neuropsychologist to develop a more specific set of academic accommodations, and give Sally more detailed strategies that will allow her to continue her schoolwork while she is recovering.

Over the next few weeks Sally starts taking the melatonin. She notes that she is able to fall asleep more easily when she goes to bed at night. However, she often wakes up after only five or six hours of sleep and is unable to return to sleep. While her headaches are occurring less often and less intensely than they were prior to starting melatonin, they are still quite bothersome, particularly at the end of the school day. She returns to see the concussion specialist to discuss the results of her MRI as well as her EKG. When she reports that she is still having some difficulty with sleep and her headaches are still interfering with her ability to complete the school day, he offers her trial of amitriptyline.

Amitriptyline, he explains, is a medication that was initially used to treat depression. However, over the years, doctors have noticed that patients who suffer from migraine headaches often have some relief of the headaches while taking amitriptyline. Their migraines occur less frequently, and are less painful, when migraine sufferers take amitriptyline. Over time, this medication became a therapy for headaches in general. Ultimately, it was prescribed for people suffering from post-concussive headaches. Patients who are suffering from post-concussive headaches report that when they start taking amitriptyline, their headaches occur less frequently. When their headaches do occur, they are less intense. In addition, amitriptyline is such a powerful medicine for treating headaches that often only one-tenth of the dose used to treat depression is necessary in order to reduce headaches. At such a small dose, side effects are rare. The most common side effect is sleepiness or drowsiness. Since many patients suffering from concussion have insomnia, just like Sally, this side effect is often desirable.

The MRI report states that Sally's brain is normal, suggesting that her symptoms are due to a concussion alone, as opposed to some other reason. Since her EKG was also normal, Sally is a candidate for taking amitriptyline. After a discussion with the concussion specialist about the risks and benefits of amitriptyline, Sally and her mother decide this is a medicine Sally should try. Therefore, she is prescribed a very low dose. The doctor recommends she take it only at night, just as she is getting into bed. Although she may not notice improvement in her headaches until she has been on the medication for several days, she will notice the sleepiness even the first night she takes it. He explains the medicine is not used to treat headaches after they start. Rather, amitriptyline prevents headaches from occurring in the first place. Therefore, he asks that Sally take it every night, even if she is doing well, without a headache. The goal is to reduce the frequency with which she gets headaches and reduce the intensity of her headaches during the daytime. If, at the end of three weeks of taking the amitriptyline nightly, Sally has not noticed a significant improvement in her headaches or insomnia, he recommends she double the dose. He schedules a follow-up appointment in six weeks' time.

Sally begins taking the amitriptyline nightly. After being on the medication for a few weeks, she notices significant improvement in her sleep. She is able to fall asleep readily. She is able to sleep through the night, often achieving eight to nine hours of sleep per evening. She has also had improvement in her headaches. They are occurring much less frequently. She's getting them only three to four times a week, most often after a long school day or a significant amount of studying. When the headaches do occur, they are much less intense than they were previously. When they are at their worst, she rates them a two on a scale of 0 to 6.

When Sally has her appointment with the neuropsychologist, she reports that she has had improvement in her sleep and headaches. However, she still notices that she is having difficulty with her schoolwork. Specifically, she finds that her nightly homework assignments take her three to four hours to complete, even though she is only taking four classes as opposed to her usual seven classes. She reports that prior to her concussion, she was able to complete her evening homework for all seven classes in approximately two and half hours. She still notices that she needs to read sentences multiple times over before she can understand them completely. She notes that her memory is poor. She finds it difficult studying for tests and quizzes. She is only able to hold on to information for a short period of time.

She spends several hours with the neuropsychologist. He uses multiple games, puzzles, tasks, and tests to assess her brain function. Some of these are computerized. Others involve cards, pencils, and paper. At the end of the assessment he informs Sally and her mother that her cognitive abilities have been affected by her concussion. He reports that she is unable to do tasks that, given her previous academic record, she was likely able to do very readily prior to her injury. He reports that she will regain all of her previous brain function, but that it may take some time. He writes her a more specific and detailed academic plan for her to bring to her school and give to her teachers, school counselor, and principle. He again emphasizes the need for full physical rest. He reviews the need for cognitive rest, with the exception of the work she is doing for school. He tells Sally and her mother that he will send a report to the physician managing her concussion.

When Sally once again follows up with the concussion specialist, she reports that she has not had any headaches for the previous 10 days. Both she and her mother have noticed a significant improvement in her overall mood. She is still complaining of difficulty with school, however. She is wondering if she can start exercising again.

The report from the neuropsychologist shows that Sally still has significant deficits in her brain function. Before her injury she was academically very high achieving. Now, her brain function is worse than 85 percent of the other female high school students her age throughout the country. This, he explains, is the likely reason for the decrease in her grades.

Given that Sally is no longer having headaches or insomnia, the concussion specialist recommends she stop taking the amitriptyline. He does inform Sally and her mother that she may have a recurrence of her headaches for the first few days after stopping the amitriptyline. However, if she is able to tolerate them, she should continue to stay off of the medication. These will likely resolve over a few days. If she wishes, she may engage in some light aerobic activity, as long as it does not make her symptoms worse. He recommends stationary bicycling as a safe way to get some light aerobic activity. If it does make her symptoms worse she should return to full physical rest. If it does not increase her symptoms, she may continue to do aerobic activity, with the understanding that she should stop if it makes her symptoms worse.

With regard to her difficulty remembering, difficulty concentrating, poor grades, and poor neuropsychological test scores, the concussion specialist discusses some possible medications with Sally and her mother. He informs them both that the medications are somewhat experimental. There are some medical studies that suggest patients who suffer a traumatic brain injury may have improvement in their brain function if given these medications. He also informs them, however, that some medical studies show no improvement in brain function in patients taking these medications. As with all medications, there are some side effects associated with these medications. They act directly on the nerve cells of the brain, or neurons. He discusses with them, in detail, some other potential reactions. However, since Sally has been suffering from post-concussive symptoms for so long and the symptoms have had such a negative impact on her quality of life and academic performance, he does think it would be reasonable to consider starting one of these medications.

After a long conversation, Sally and her mother decide not to take any experimental medications at this time. She has improved so significantly over the last several weeks that they hope she will regain all of her brain function relatively soon. They also hope that many of her other symptoms, such as decreased energy, feeling depressed, and irritability, will improve when she is allowed to exercise. Therefore, they will continue with their current plan. If, however, she has not improved at the time of the next follow-up appointment, they may reconsider these medications. They make a plan to follow up with the concussion specialist again in six to eight weeks.

Two months later Sally follows up with the concussion specialist. She reports that overall she feels completely recovered. She has had a significant improvement in her memory, concentration, mood, energy level, and all other symptoms. At that appointment she rates her post-concussion symptom scale score a total of zero. She reports that she has been able to improve her grades, scoring an A on her last math test and a B plus in biology.

She brings with her the results from her follow up appointment with the neuropsychologist. The report shows that Sally had a marked improvement in her scores. Her memory is currently better than 97 percent of other girls her age throughout the country. Her reaction time, processing speed, and all other measurements of her brain function are better than 88 percent of other girls her age throughout the country. The neuropsychologist believes that Sally has improved and is perhaps completely recovered. However, he does want to see her one final time before she is cleared to return to contact sports. The point of that visit will be to obtain one final measurement of her brain function that might serve as a baseline or standard assessment of her brain function in the unfortunate event of another concussion in the future.

The concussion specialist is pleased by this news. He recommends that Sally gradually return to a full academic load. He asks that she work with her school and school teachers to determine the best way to return her to all seven classes. She should develop a plan, with the school, to make up any work that she missed during her recovery. He also allows Sally to gradually start returning to sport. Since her last visit, she has been exercising 4 to 5 days a week for 20 to 30 minutes on the stationary bicycle. She reports she has only been doing some light to moderate cycling. She is hoping to run track this spring. In preparation for track season, he recommends she start advancing her aerobic activity by jogging. If after a week of jogging relatively short distances at a moderate pace she remains symptom-free, he recommends Sally start jogging longer distances and add on some sprinting. If she is able to run longer distances and sprint without any return of her symptoms, he recommends adding on some resistance training, such as push-ups, sit-ups, or weight lifting. If she is able to tolerate this as well, she may start practicing with the track team. He gives her some guidelines to help guide her along return-to-play stages he has just described. He recommends that her athletic trainer help her through the stages. He insists that she avoid any activities that place her at an increased risk of contact to the head. He will see her again in approximately six weeks, which is just prior to the start of the track season.

Over the following weeks Sally works closely with her athletic trainer. Under the guidance of the athletic trainer, she gradually returns to sport specific activities. Ultimately, she is able to run five miles in a day without any recurrence of her symptoms. She is able to do 50-yard sprints. She has even started throwing the javelin. She has been doing push-ups and sit-ups, as well as some resistance training in the weight room. None of these activities have resulted in a recurrence of her symptoms.

With regard to her schoolwork, Sally has been able to add on the three classes she had dropped earlier in the year. Her teachers were understanding of her injury. They offered to combine Sally's grades before and after her injury and to use these as her grades for the year. They did not require her to make up any additional reading assignments that she missed during her absence.

There were, however, some key aspects of American history that Sally missed and her teachers felt were important for her to learn prior to graduation. They were able to work out a plan where Sally could make up some of these missed assignments, and receive some extra tutoring on the weekends, which helped her make up some of the homework she had missed.

When she followed up for her next appointment with the concussion specialist, Sally looked like a new person. She was all smiles. Her energy was back. Her mood was back. Her mother reported, "This is the daughter I know." She told her doctor that she was able to perform all athletic activities without any recurrence of her symptoms. She was now enrolled in a full academic schedule, taking all seven classes. She did not have any symptoms, despite doing all of her homework and much of the makeup work. She had been to see the neuropsychologist, where she had further measurements taken of her brain function. The report showed that she scored higher than 90 percent of other girls her age throughout the country in every category. The neuropsychologist said that these could be used as a baseline in the future, if necessary. Sally was anxious to return to athletics, and live her life fully again, without restrictions.

As she has been completely symptom-free for the last six weeks, including with full physical exertion and full cognitive exertion, the concussion specialist believes that Sally is completely recovered from her injury. Her neuropsychologist agrees, and reports that her most recent cognitive scores are consistent with complete recovery and consistent with her previous performance. Her athletic trainer agrees that Sally has been able to perform well in athletics without any apparent recurrence of her symptoms. Therefore, the concussion specialist has Sally perform a baseline symptom inventory, which reveals a zero for all symptoms typical of concussion. As noted, she has had a computerized neuropsychological baseline assessment performed by her neuropsychologist. The concussion specialist performs a balance error system score to serve as a baseline in her future. She is cleared for full participation in athletics without any restrictions. He reminds Sally that should she experience any recurrence of her symptoms or new injuries when she returns to contact during soccer season next fall, she must immediately report to her athletic trainer or doctor. When she returns to school, her athletic trainer repeats a sideline assessment of concussion. She will repeat this again in the fall prior to start of soccer season but wanted to obtain a baseline sideline assessment now in case of unexpected injury before the start of the next soccer season.

Sally's case illustrates a more complicated concussion recovery. There are several points worth making about it.

1. Sally is not instructed to rest completely immediately after her injury. It is likely, that by continuing to exercise before she was completely recovered from her concussion, Sally unknowingly delayed her recovery. Had she been instructed early on to rest completely, she may have recovered more quickly.

2. Sally continued to read, do her homework, and perform other cognitive tasks after her injury. This, too, likely delayed her recovery. Had she been instructed to obtain full cognitive rest soon after her injury, she may have recovered more quickly.

3. Most of the physicians involved in Sally's care soon after her concussion recommended she wait "a week," after her injury or "a week after her symptoms resolve," prior to returning to athletics. This was one of the standard recommendations not too long ago. But recently, this approach has changed in light of new medical evidence. Many primary care physicians, internists, pediatricians, neurologists, and other clinicians will be well aware of the new recommendations for managing concussions and will be true experts in caring for concussed athletes. However, since the assessment and management of concussed athletes has changed so much in the last several years, many will be unfamiliar with the new recommendations. Concussed athletes should see their primary care physicians after a concussive brain injury. If their physician is uncomfortable managing concussions, he or she will usually know of a doctor who specializes in this area that they can refer athletes to.

4. Sally is offered some experimental medications that she chooses not to take. In medicine, there are always more options. There are always other treatments or therapies that can be tried. But each athlete must weigh the likelihood of benefit of these treatments against the potential for adverse effects. If the symptoms of a concussion are tolerable, it is often best to allow them to heal naturally, as opposed to treating them with medications. However, for those athletes whose symptoms are negatively impacting their quality of life, these medications are a safe and reasonable option.

In summary, the ideal concussion program involves many clinicians in various specialties, all working together to care for concussed athletes. The best concussion management plans start before the athlete ever takes to the field, court, or ice, by obtaining baseline measurements. Identifying medical providers with an interest in managing athletes who sustain concussions is the first step in trying to organize a concussion management program. For clinicians working with a given team, school, or other group of athletes, a written concussion action plan can help ensure that athletes receive the best possible care.

SUGGESTED READINGS

Lovell, M. R., R. E. Echemendia, J. T. Barth, and M. W. Collins, *Traumatic Brain Injury in Sports: An International Neuropsychological Perspective.* 2004, Lisse, The Netherlands: Swets and Zeitlinger.

McCrea, M., *Mild Traumatic Brain Injury and Postconcussion Syndrome: The New Evidence Base for Diagnosis and Treatment.* 2008, New York: Oxford University Press.

14

THE FUTURE: WHAT MEDICAL RESEARCH MAY LEAD TO IN THE FUTURE

When it comes to athletes sustaining concussions in sports, many unanswered questions remain:

a. Is there a genetic predisposition to concussion, and can athletes be tested for it?
b. Is there a medication that might effectively treat concussive brain injury, as opposed to only treating the symptoms?
c. Is there a medication that can prevent the cumulative effects of concussions?
d. Is there a blood test that might be used to determine when an athlete has sustained a concussion or when an athlete has completely recovered from a concussion?
e. Is there a type of imaging that can allow doctors to "see" a concussion?

Future medical and scientific research will seek to answer these questions. These efforts will likely focus on:

- Discovering more about what happens to the brain when an athlete is concussed.
- Discovering whether or not certain athletes are predisposed to sustaining concussions or predisposed to bad outcomes after sustaining multiple sport-related concussions.
- Discovering how we can more accurately diagnose a sport-related concussion, determining both when in fact an athlete's symptoms are attributable to a sport-related concussion and determining precisely when the athlete has recovered completely from his or her sport-related concussion.
- Discovering potential treatments that will assist athletes in recovering from sport-related concussions, helping them recover faster, and helping them prevent any long-term problems.

Some of the most recent medical studies are discussed below.

ACCELEROMETERS

One of the newest technologies used to investigate sport-related concussions uses a device known as an accelerometer. Accelerometers are small sensors that are placed into the helmets of athletes during practice or competition. These sensors can be used to measure the amount of force of a given impact. They can measure the speed and direction a helmet moves after impact. They record how fast and in what direction the helmet spins after an impact. These measurements can then be correlated to athletes who sustain a sport-related concussion. The characteristics of the impacts causing sport-related concussions can be compared to those impacts that do not result in a sport-related concussion. These data might help us understand more about what exactly it is that leads to concussive brain injury.

Preliminary data using these sensors has revealed that concussion occur after a wide range of forces, resulting in a wide range of accelerations. Symptoms do not necessarily correlate with the amount of force involved in the impact, or with the maximum acceleration produced by the impact. This suggests that other factors play a significant part in determining whether or not a concussion occurs and how long it takes to recover from a concussion.

PREDISPOSITION

Some athletes may be predisposed to concussion, meaning they may be more likely to suffer a sport-related concussion than other athletes. Similarly, some athletes, while they may not be more likely to sustain sport-related concussions, may be more vulnerable to the effects of concussions. They may be more likely than other athletes to suffer long-term problems after sustaining multiple concussions. They may suffer more diminished cognitive function after sustaining concussions. They may suffer from longer recovery times than other athletes. The ability to identify these athletes could be used to prevent injuries.

For example, if there was a test that could determine which athletes are more likely to sustain sport-related concussions, athletes could be screened prior to participating in high-risk sports. Those who tested positive, and therefore knew that they were more vulnerable to sustaining a sport-related concussion, might choose to participate in safer sports, such as swimming, rather than higher risk sports such as football and ice hockey. Another option would be to test only those athletes who had sustained at least one sport-related concussion. Those, who after sustaining their first sport-related concussion were found to be at increased risk compared to other athletes, might choose not to play high-risk sports. Those who underwent the test and were not found to be at increased risk of sustaining sport-related concussions might chose to continue playing.

Similarly, if physicians could predict which athletes were more likely to suffer a bad outcome after sustaining a sport-related concussion or multiple concussions, they could use this information to help athletes decide whether or not to continue playing high-risk contact or collision sports. Efforts have been made to identify just such a test.

Some medical studies indicate that certain athletes may have a genetic predisposition to poor outcome after sustaining a concussion, multiple concussions, or even multiple repeated blows to the head that do not cause concussions. The most well studied gene is known as apolipoprotein E epsilon 4, or "APOE4" for short. Some of the earliest medical literature to study APOE4 was performed in boxers. A physician named Barry Jordan assessed neurological status of multiple retired boxers. He noted that those who carried this particular gene, APOE4, had worse brain function than those who did not. Boxers who had fought in more bouts, and were therefore exposed to a greater number of blows to the head, had worse brain function than those boxers who fought in less bouts over their careers. Those boxers who carried the APOE4 gene *and* fought in a high number of bouts, had the worst brain function.

Other medical studies, conducted outside of the realm of athletics, suggest that people who carry this particular gene and who also sustain a concussion or other traumatic brain injury at some point during their lifetime are at increased risk of poor outcomes, including an increased risk of Alzheimer's disease.

These studies are preliminary, however. The effects of carrying APOE4 on neurological function after brain injury are poorly understood. Some studies show that APOE4 has no effect on outcome after sustainment of head injury. In fact, in some patients, having the APOE4 gene may be beneficial. APOE4 may be beneficial for children who sustain an injury to the brain. Combined, these studies suggest that the effects of APOE4 after a traumatic brain injury may be different depending on how old a person is at the time of injury.

In order to help further understand the role age may play in determining the effects of APOE4 after traumatic brain injury, investigators have taken to the laboratory. One of my colleagues, Rebekah Mannix, M.D., conducted an experiment in mice that was published in the *Journal of Cerebral Blood Flow and Metabolism*. Some of the mice had the APOE4 gene, others did not. All mice underwent a traumatic brain injury. Adult mice that had the APOE4 gene had worse brain function after injury than mice without the APOE4 gene. However, immature or "pediatric" mice with the APOE4 gene had the same brain function after injury as mice without the APOE4 gene. The results suggest that the APOE4 gene may have harmful effects for adult mice who sustain a traumatic brain injury, while in pediatric mice that sustain a traumatic brain injury the gene may have no effect. Experiments continue to try and determine exactly what APOE4 does after brain injury that seems to effect outcome, and why the effects seem to be different based on the age at the time of injury.

These experiments are exciting. They offer hope, that one day we may be able to predict which athletes are at risk for poor outcomes after a concussion. *However, until we learn more about APOE, its function after brain injury, whether or not the results are consistent, and how age affects outcome, it cannot be used clinically to treat athletes. Currently, APOE4 is not a useful test, and should not be measured in patients, athletes or otherwise, for the purpose of trying to assess outcome after traumatic brain injury.*

MARKERS OF INJURY

In addition to genes, researchers have also searched for blood tests that might be associated with concussive brain injury or brain function after injury and perhaps used to monitor recovery from injury. "Serum markers" are proteins, chemicals, or other molecules in the blood that can be used to identify a certain disease or disease process. Two of the most commonly discussed serum markers that have been investigated for the assessment of concussive brain injury are the "S-100B" protein and "neuron specific enolase" (NSE). In a study out of Germany published in 2001 in the *Journal of Neurology, Neurosurgery and Psychiatry*, Herrmann and colleagues measured S-100B and NSE in patients who had sustained traumatic brain injuries, mostly concussions. Both serum markers, S-100b and NSE, were measured on the first, second, and third days after injury. Patients had their brain function measured two weeks after admission to the hospital and again six months later. Those patients who had more S-100B and NSE in their blood after injury had worse brain function, both in the tests performed soon after injury, and those performed six months later. These finding suggest that these two serum markers might prove useful in determining which athletes will suffer significant and prolonged losses of brain function after concussion. Other studies have also found that theses serum markers may be useful in identifying patients who have sustained a traumatic brain injury, or in identifying those at risk for prolonged recovery after injury.

However, these findings have not been consistent. Some studies have failed to reveal any utility in testing for S-100B or NSE. Some studies show elevations in these serum markers in patients without brain injury. This suggests that there may be other reasons why these markers are elevated. Until further research has been conducted, neither of these serum markers can be used clinically, to assess and treat patients, with reliability.

Other factors, have also been studies as potentially leading to poor outcomes after concussion. In particular, researchers have investigated whether or not athletes who experience certain symptoms after their concussion have larger deficits in brain function or take longer to recover. A study performed at the University of Pittsburgh and led by neuropsychologist Micky Collins that was published in the *American Journal of Sports Medicine* in 2003, separated athletes who sustained a concussion into two groups: 1) those reporting a headache one week after their injury, and 2) those without a headache after the same interval. Their results showed that those athletes still reporting a headache one week after injury had worse memory and slower reaction times than those athletes not reporting a headache. The study also found that athletes reporting headaches were more likely to have suffered amnesia at the time of their injury. An additional study by many of the same investigators showed that athletes who suffered migraine headache symptoms after their concussions took longer to recover from their injuries than those athletes who did not report migraine headache–type symptoms.

This correlation, between headaches—migraine headaches in particular—and recovery from concussion led some researchers to wonder whether athletes who have suffered from migraine headaches in the past might be at increased risk of sustaining a concussion. Indeed, a study out of Canada, published in the *British Journal of Sports Medicine* in 2006, analyzed data collected by the Canadian Community Health Survey. Those athletes who were diagnosed as having migraine headaches by a health professional were more likely to have sustained a sport-related concussion in the previous 12 months than those athletes not diagnosed with migraines. Currently, a joint study between Children's Hospital Boston and the University of Pittsburgh is analyzing the effects of migraines on recovery from sport-related concussion.

Headaches and migraines in particular are not the only symptoms being investigated as possible determinants of sport-related concussion recovery. After sustaining a concussion, many athletes will complain of feeling "in a fog." This is a subjective symptom, meaning it cannot be easily measured or quantified. Although many athletes use this term, and have an inherent understanding of its meaning, it is difficult to define. Still, several clinicians have observed associations between this symptom, "fogginess," and poor outcome after sport-related concussion. A study published in the *Journal of the International Neuropsychological Society* in 2004, measured overall concussion symptoms and neuropsychological test scores of athletes who reported feeling foggy, and compared the findings to athletes who did not report feeling foggy. Athletes who reported fogginess experienced a larger number of other post-concussion symptoms than those not reporting fogginess. Furthermore, athletes who reported feeling foggy had slower reaction times, worse memory, and took more time to complete neurocognitive tasks than athletes not reporting fogginess.

Many other factors are being considered as potentially increasing an athlete's risk of either sustaining a concussion, suffering a long recovery after a concussion, or suffering long-term effects later in life after sustaining a concussion or multiple concussions earlier in life. Other illnesses or diseases such as attention deficit/hyperactivity disorder, post-traumatic stress disorder, anxiety and depression are all being investigated currently. Perhaps certain medications that athletes are taking at the time of their injury may protect against the effects of concussion, or worsen the outcome after concussion. The shape of the skull, musculature of the neck and shoulders, or other anatomic considerations may affect one's risk of concussion or recovery from concussion. Studies to look for these potential risk factors will hopefully lead to a better understanding of which athletes are at greatest risk.

IMAGING

Earlier in this book we learned that pictures of the brain, such as computed tomograms of the head (head CTs) or magnetic resonance images (MRIs), appear normal in athletes who have sustained concussions. But there are other types of pictures available. Some investigators seek to discover ways of picturing or imaging the brain that can allow us to "see" a concussion in an injured athlete. Several such methods of imaging have been studied.

Functional MRI (fMRI)

Functional MRI is somewhat complicated to explain. Perhaps the easiest way to think about it is as a picture of the brain that allows doctors to see which parts of the brain are in use, receiving increased amounts of blood flow, while the patient is completing certain tasks. In other words, an athlete who is undergoing an fMRI after a concussion is asked to complete certain mathematical tasks. While the athlete completes these tasks, images or pictures are taken of the brain. These pictures show various parts of the brain lit up in different colors, based on how vigorously that part of the brain is being used, and how much blood flow that part of the brain is receiving. It allows doctors to see which part of the brain is "activated" and how hard a given part of the brain is working.

Studies have shown that athletes who have sustained sport-related concussions use different parts of the brain to a higher degree than athletes who are not concussed. In addition, as athletes recover from their concussions, and regain their previous levels of brain functioning, the changes in their fMRIs go away. Once athletes have recovered, their fMRIs look similar to those of athletes who have not sustained a concussion.

Diffusion Tensor Imaging (DTI)

DTI is another variation on traditional MRI scanning. Again, DTI can be somewhat difficult to understand for readers without scientific or medical training. Perhaps the easiest way to think about it is as a picture or image of the brain that allows doctors to see the movement of water in the brain. Recall earlier in the book when we discussed the cells of the brain known as neurons. Each neuron had a long, narrow section known as the axon. Well, water inside of a neuron can travel down the length of the axon. But it can also travel perpendicular to the axon, across the cell membrane. Doctors can detect certain changes in the brain cells by measuring the direction in which the water of the brain is traveling. Studies in children and adolescents after concussive brain injury have shown abnormal DTIs of the brain, even though CT scans and traditional MRIs appear normal. Thus, DTI may help diagnose a concussion, even though the more traditional forms of brain imaging show normal results.

TREATMENTS

Currently, there are no known effective treatments for traumatic brain injury. Physicians provide "supportive care" for patients with major injuries. These patients are often comatose, or have such pronounced brain dysfunction that they cannot think clearly. "Supportive care" means that doctors help the patients breathe, maintain blood pressure, relieve pressure build-up in the brain due to swelling or bleeding, provide nutrition, and basically, keep patients alive until they are able to recover from the injury on their own.

For patients with milder injury, as is more common for athletes, we can treat some of the symptoms of concussion. Therapies like the physical and cognitive rest discussed previously, help to treat many of the symptoms. Academic accommodations can be used to help athletes obtain cognitive rest while in school. Some medications can be used to treat headaches, insomnia, poor cognitive function, and other specific symptoms of concussion. But ultimately, there is no direct treatment for the concussion itself, no treatment that helps athletes recover faster. Discovering such a treatment is the main goal of many of us currently caring for concussed athletes.

There are several potential options.

Three years ago, I attended a lecture given by Michael Whalen, M.D. Dr. Whalen is the head of a laboratory in the neuroscience center of the Massachusetts General Hospital that investigates traumatic brain injury. I approached him about developing a model of concussion that would allow us to study potential therapies. Since that time, we have developed models of severe, moderate, and mild concussive brain injuries. These models can now be used to test potential treatments. In fact, by using these models, we have found a molecule that spares the loss of cognitive function after traumatic brain injury.

SUGGESTED READINGS

Anderson, R. E., et al., High Serum S100B Levels for Trauma Patients Without Head Injuries. *Neurosurgery,* 2001. 48(6): 1255–58; discussion 1258–60.

Biberthaler, P., et al., Serum S-100B Concentration Provides Additional Information for the Indication of Computed Tomography in Patients after Minor Head Injury: A Prospective Multicenter Study. *Shock,* 2006. 25(5): 446–53.

Chen, J. K., et al., A Validation of the Post Concussion Symptom Scale in the Assessment of Complex Concussion Using Cognitive Testing and Functional MRI. *J Neurol Neurosurg Psychiatry,* 2007. 78(11): 1231–38.

Collins, M. W., et al., Relationship between Postconcussion Headache and Neuropsychological Test Performance in High School Athletes. *Am J Sports Med,* 2003. 31(2): 168–73.

de Kruijk, J. R., et al., S-100B and Neuron-Specific Enolase in Serum of Mild Traumatic Brain Injury Patients. A Comparison with Health Controls. *Acta Neurol Scand,* 2001. 103(3): 175–79.

Guskiewicz, K. M., et al., Measurement of Head Impacts in Collegiate Football Players: Relationship between Head Impact Biomechanics and Acute Clinical Outcome after Concussion. *Neurosurgery,* 2007. 61(6): 1244–52; discussion 1252–53.

Iverson, G. L., et al., Relation between Subjective Fogginess and Neuropsychological Testing Following Concussion. *J Int Neuropsychol Soc,* 2004. 10(6): 904–6.

Jordan, B. D., et al., Apolipoprotein E Epsilon4 Associated with Chronic Traumatic Brain Injury in Boxing. *JAMA,* 1997. 278(2): 136–40.

Khuman, J. et al., Tumor Necrosis Factor Alpha and Fas Receptor Contribute to Cognitive Deficits Independent of Cell Death after Concussive Traumatic Brain Injury in Mice. *J Cereb Blood Flow Metab,* 2010. epub ahead of print.

Liberman, J. N., et al., Apolipoprotein E Epsilon 4 and Short-Term Recovery from Predominantly Mild Brain Injury. *Neurology,* 2002. 58(7): 1038–44.

Linstedt, U., et al., Serum Concentration of S-100 Protein in Assessment of Cognitive Dysfunction after General Anesthesia in Different Types of Surgery. *Acta Anaesthesiol Scand,* 2002. 46(4): 384–89.

Mannix, R. C., et al., Age-Dependent Effect of Apolipoprotein E4 on Functional Outcome after Controlled Cortical Impact in Mice. *J Cereb Blood Flow Metab,* 2011. 31(1): 351–61.

Mayeux, R., et al., Synergistic Effects of Traumatic Head Injury and Apolipoprotein-Epsilon 4 in Patients with Alzheimer's Disease. *Neurology,* 1995. 45(3 Pt 1): 555–57.

Pelinka, L. E., et al., Circulating S100B Is Increased after Bilateral Femur Fracture Without Brain Injury in the Rat. *Br J Anaesth,* 2003. 91(4): 595–97.

Teasdale, G. M., et al., Association of Apolipoprotein E Polymorphism with Outcome after Head Injury. *Lancet,* 1997. 350(9084): 1069–71.

15

In Their Own Words: Athletes from the Sports Concussion Clinic of Children's Hospital Boston

Since cofounding the Sports Concussion Clinic in the Division of Sports Medicine at Children's Hospital Boston in 2007, I have been privileged to care for some wonderful young athletes. Fortunately, many have recovered quickly, without complications. But others have suffered through long, frustrating recoveries. Some were plagued by repetitive head injuries, despite refraining from contact and collision sports. For some, their injuries changed their lives, their network of friends, and their academic performance. I can think of no better way to conclude this book than to have three exceptional athletes describe their own experiences with concussions and relay to the readers how their injuries affected their lives.

Maggie Hickey

Heading into October of my sophomore year of high school, I was pretty typical. I had a fun group of friends. I was a good student. I was looking forward to another great season of rowing on the crew team. I was excited to no longer be a lowly freshman and entered the school with confidence on the first day. The teachers I had were going to be challenging, but I had always been able to maintain good grades. So keeping up with academics never entered my mind.

On October 3, 2008, everything I knew to be my life began to unravel. It was a Friday. My friends and I had planned to go to the football game. We were getting ready at a friend's house. I remember not feeling well. I called my mom to come and get me. Before she could drive the mile between our house and my friend's she got a call from my friend's mother telling her that I had fainted and had a gash on my head. Although I had passed out, they had been able to wake me up. My friends found me on the stone floor on the way to the bathroom, apparently having hit my head on the doorknob as I went down. When I woke up, I was disoriented and didn't remember what had happened. After a trip to the emergency room I came home with stitches that went through my eyebrow. I had a normal CAT scan of my brain. So the biggest worry I had was covering up the stitches, and hoping there was not a large scar remaining once it healed. I don't remember calling my mom before I fainted. I figured the memory loss probably meant I hit my head pretty hard. The ER staff recommended that my parents wake me up periodically that night, "just in case I had a concussion." But other than that I was fine. I was acting normally and we were sent on our way.

The next day we had a regatta and the ER staff had cleared me to row if the stitches weren't bothering me. I chose to sit out because I had been up really late the night before, and my headache had not subsided. I was committed to rowing, and was looking forward to a strong season. So by Tuesday I was back at practice, running, using the ergometer machines, and on the water rowing. But I began to have debilitating headaches from exercising, reading, and being in the sunlight. I started having trouble finding homework papers. I forgot my books for class. I was chronically exhausted. At home, I hoped to sleep. But my headaches were so bad, and I was so queasy by the end of the day, that I wasn't' able to put my head down. I had been raised to muscle through. So for a while I would just take Motrin, and hope the pain would go away and not come back. I missed a few practices. But for the most part, during the first three weeks after the injury, I tried as hard as I could to maintain my normal schedule. During that time, school became extremely difficult. The lights at the school caused me to get headaches. My eyes were so sensitive it was difficult to keep them open. The noise confused me, although I don't think I recognized it as confusion at the time. I was scattered, and not able to keep my work organized. I had been an avid reader, and now, could not read a page without difficulty. I was exhausted and in a constant state of "headache."

My mother says that physically I became nearly unrecognizable to her. My eyes were barely able to open, my skin color was off. I was dragging through my days. The constant nausea made it hard to eat anything. I began to sink deeper into a dazed trance. I went to the pediatrician twice during the first three weeks. Each time we came home having been told to take it easy. On the third visit, my pediatrician, who has known me since I was seven years old, could see the changes in my face. She sent me immediately to the emergency room. They ran a few tests and hooked me up to an IV to try to end the headache in hopes that if they could stop the cycle my headaches would end altogether. However, the medication they gave me caused an allergic reaction. So, it only made things worse. After realizing that nothing was working, the hospital referred me to a local doctor that tested for concussions. The studies that were done later that week showed that I had a pretty severe concussion. I scored less than the first percentile on one of the tests, and not much better on the rest. So finally, weeks after the injury we knew why I was having so much trouble doing the things that had been so easy for me before my concussion. I was given a few weeks to go easy at school. Half days were suggested. Exercise stopped completely. I was told if I felt better in a few weeks to redo the concussion test. I did take a second test. When this one wasn't any better, I was referred up to Children's Hospital Boston, and Dr. Meehan.

By the time I was in to see Dr. Meehan, it was just before Christmas. I had spent a month navigating my schoolwork. I had missed a few days after the initial testing came back. I went back to school as soon as I felt a little better. As soon as I was back in the school, the symptoms would kick in again. I couldn't do the smallest amount of homework. I couldn't read one page, let along three chapters. I was frustrated and getting worried. I remember other kids in school with concussions, and how everyone would say they were fine. The other students would gossip talk about them, complaining about how they got to skip a test because they said they had a "concussion." I didn't want to be the kid that people were talking about. So I tried to keep up with everything: taking tests I wasn't ready for, trying to read for all of my classes, staying after school for extra math help. I took a lot of half days, but tried to stay in school as much as I could. I wasn't rowing. So I had time to regroup after school. But often, by the time I came home, my headaches were crippling. I cried a lot, wondering when I'd feel better and asking my mother why I wasn't getting better. Keeping up with everything was too overwhelming. I wasn't resting enough to help my symptoms. During this time the headaches were never-ending. It was becoming too much to handle. Then we went to Dr. Meehan, and the healing began.

Dr. Meehan told me to put my brain on rest. He helped me understand that, ultimately, I would heal and feel better. But it would take time and patience. We needed to manage my brain activity, and the best way for that to happen would be to shut my brain down for a while. I was told to cut my schoolwork down to a minimum, avoid crew practice, and take it easy with regards to my social life. That's not particularly easy for a 16-year-old student and athlete. But I felt great relief knowing that I would ultimately be back to normal. I tried not to feel sorry for myself while my family was skiing every day over winter break, or that my friends were together, or that I couldn't read. I watched a full season of *One Tree Hill* and watched a ton of other movies and television shows. I had trouble on the computer. So I couldn't use that too much. For a solid two-week period my parents and doctor insisted I do nothing. Sounds like a dream, but it was more of a nightmare. It's hard to shut down like that when you're not used to it. I had high hopes that if I did truly shut down, then after two weeks this would all be over. That wasn't how it would go for me. But it became clear that the less my brain did, the fewer symptoms I had. It wasn't until April that I would finally be symptom-free. A full six months after the fainting spell that caused the concussion.

During the three months after Christmas, we had a meeting with all of my teachers, my guidance counselor, and the school nurse to keep everyone on board with how the concussion would affect my schoolwork. We talked about the possibility of my being placed on a special education plan. It would have required that I be given more academic accommodations. As it turned out, I was not able to take advantage of this because I had compensated so well. I managed to keep my grades above the need for concern. That was by the school's standards, not my standards or those of my parents. My straight A's were becoming C's. And there were tons of assignments that were incomplete. I could only manage half of a regular school day, and could only do part of most assignments. I was still expected, at some point, to get everything done. The nurse at the meeting made sure I understood that if I needed a break, there was a place for me in her office. I appreciated that everyone was willing to be patient, and did their best to accommodate me. But the reality was that I was still responsible for a lot of work that I was unable to do.

I don't like to have attention drawn to me. I was very uncomfortable being in the classroom when everyone else was taking a test or presenting a project that I wasn't participating in. I perceived that my peers thought I should be done with my symptoms and back to normal, that I was somehow using the concussion as a continued excuse to not have to do the work. Actually I would have given anything to be able to complete the work. My close friends would joke about how I "got out of going to school," or how I "conveniently" couldn't take a test. I found myself asking to miss the classes when I knew they would be working on something I hadn't completed yet. I didn't want to be singled out as a kid that people think is taking the easy way out. I felt that the only accommodation my teachers had given was more time to complete the same amount of work. They put it all back on me to navigate my way through the work. They often said, "Do what you can." Well, what I could do and what was actually necessary for me to do were two different things. I remember having a poem to memorize in English. After struggling for 40 minutes with the first line, my mother told me to put it away. She insisted that I no longer try to memorize it, and tell the teacher that I couldn't. It was hard, but in retrospect I wish I'd had the courage to do that more often. My knowledge on subjects could have been assessed with a lot less work. Half of the math problems for homework might have been sufficient. But I didn't reach out for that help. If it was assigned, I did it. Sometimes slowly, mostly late, but it got done. Dr. Meehan gave the analogy that if someone had a broken arm, they wouldn't be required to do push-ups in gym class. They would be obviously injured, and temporarily incapable of doing push-ups until they recovered. He said it's the same for a concussion and an academic class. The few times I reluctantly agreed to miss things, it was because my parents insisted or intervened with a teacher.

I remember one day in February I went to the nurse's office for Motrin. She wouldn't give it to me, because I told her I had taken some earlier that morning. I was sent away. Remember that a member of the Health Office was at the meeting with the guidance counsellor and my teachers. They had repeatedly offered the Health Office as a place to go for relief. But evidently this nurse was unaware of my condition. I texted my mom and told her about the nurse's reaction. She was on the phone in minutes. But she too got attitude from the nurse, who said that my injury was months ago, and I should have only had symptoms for two weeks at most. She went on to say that we were now months later, and any headaches couldn't be from the concussion. Well, my mom handled that in a hurry with another note from Dr. Meehan saying that I was to have accommodations until he notified everyone that I had fully recovered. We had already handed in several notes just like this. But they continued to request this in writing. Bottom line, if the school nurse doesn't know how serious a concussion can be, how severe a concussion can be, and the length of time it can take to recover from a concussion, we could hardly expect the teachers and my peers to know. I wasn't aware of it until I was living it. And neither were my parents or siblings. It's not something that you wear a cast for, or use crutches to help you. So the people around you have no idea why you can't do normal daily activities.

To a certain extent my friends were beginning to realize that maybe this wasn't just a big excuse to take the easy way out. My social life screeched to a halt. I missed dances, football games, parties, and practices. I felt like I was essentially losing a year of my high school experience. My friends were going about their lives, while I was home, dealing with difficult symptoms. The few times I did try and get out for something social, even on a small scale, it would set me back. Having my friends go about their lives and enjoy high school and rowing while I sat in my house was hard for me to deal with. My concussion was holding me back in every aspect of life.

In April of 2009 I was finally free of my symptoms. I remember having my first day that was symptom-free. Then there were a few in a row. I was able to get back to my normal activities. I ran three miles the day Dr. Meehan deemed I was ready for exercise. It felt good to be able to engage in any physical activity I wanted. The good news for me was that I knew none of my symptoms were permanent. I took comfort throughout this time knowing that I would be my normal self again, although, I had plenty of periods of being impatient, unhappy about the length of my recovery. I gained an appreciation and compassion for people who need permanent accommodations at school and outside of school. I went back to rowing. I completed all of my schoolwork by the end of the school year. I was fortunate to have parents, who would advocate for me, and a doctor who was able to guide me through the healing progression. I am a senior in high school now, going through the college application process. I'm grateful for what I've been able to take away from this experience. I've become more organized and determined because of my concussion. For many of my peers it is tough juggling all that needs to be done. Applications, sports, schoolwork, SAT's all need to be completed. I became a master at prioritizing and staying organized under difficult circumstances. This is a breeze by comparison. At the time, I was worried that my trying sophomore year would affect everything in my future. Looking back now, it feels like a lifetime ago. But I will never forget what it felt like to be so affected by a concussive brain injury.

My best advice to someone going through a severe concussion is not to get too discouraged or frustrated with the time it may take to recover. It's often a long and grueling process. But things will get back to normal in time. It's not the sort of injury you can rush to heal from. So take it easy. It does get better.

Sean Folan

My name is Sean Folan. I am 17 years old and a junior at Catholic Memorial High School. For as long as I can remember, sports have been part of my life in some shape or form. I was three years old the first time my parents put a pair of skates on me and sent me off on the ice for the first time. I remember having a baseball glove that was probably bigger than me. But I tried to catch the ball anyway. I was encouraged to play all types of sports: hockey, baseball, soccer, and lacrosse. I really never could imagine that someday sports would not be a part of my day-to-day life.

I entered Catholic Memorial in seventh grade and was thrilled when I made the middle school soccer team. I remember being both excited and nervous about being at such a big school. I was excited because Catholic Memorial, or "CM" as it is often referred to, is known as a school that prides itself on having a great sports program. I wanted nothing more than to play sports for CM. The first few weeks of school were tough. Trying to figure out how I was going to go to practice every day and also get all of my homework done before I passed out from exhaustion was challenging. But somehow I figured it out. When it was time for hockey season, I had mastered what I needed to do. I looked forward to many years ahead of me involved in soccer, hockey, and baseball.

Little did I know those plans would all change for me. In a matter of three years, I suffered four concussions. The first was minor. It was followed by a second while playing hockey that left me unconscious and in the hospital for a week. I struggled with the complications that come from a serious concussion: headaches, not being able to concentrate, not being able to sleep at night, going to school, and having to go home because my head hurt too much. At times, I was just too tired to function. But with time, rest, and the great care I received at the Sports Concussion Clinic at Children's Hospital, I was eventually cleared to play hockey again.

Unfortunately, the thrill of returning to hockey would not last for long. After only being back for a couple of weeks, I again suffered a serious concussion, my third. I could not believe it. Why was this happening to me again? All I wanted was to play hockey and stay healthy. There was no mention of when I would return to sports. But I was hopeful it would happen. Six weeks later, however, while cheering on Catholic Memorial's varsity soccer team as they brought home the state championship, I fell off a fence and suffered my fourth concussion.

I was then told that, because of the number of concussions I had sustained, and the unusually long, complicated recoveries I suffered, I would never be cleared to play contact or collision sports again. WHAT?! I was only 16 years old. I went to Catholic Memorial, a school well known for its sports programs. I played sports for my town. And now, I can never play hockey, soccer, or base-ball on a team again. Needless to say it was devastating news. It is something that I still have a hard time accepting. Dr. Meehan explained the reasons behind this decision. That doctors are worried about my apparent susceptibility to injury, future damage to my brain, and other things that may affect me in the future. My parents agreed with the decision. But I can tell you that I did not. felt like I was fine and that there was nothing wrong with me. Why couldn't I play? How was I going to cope with this?

Well, I can honestly say that it has not been easy. I have been forced to face the fact that I will not be involved in sports like I have been in the past. There is not a day that goes by that I don't wish that things had gone differently for me. I miss playing sports and being part of a team. But I have to believe that this all has a purpose in my life. Hopefully, in the future, I will be involved in sports by coach-ing a team. My mother always says that things happen for a reason. When she says that, it really drives me crazy. But I believe that maybe she is right. I am still trying to figure out how I can fit sports into my life in other ways. I hope that in the future I can figure out a way to do this. These injuries have changed my life dramatically. They have forced me to live my life differently than I had expected. But I know that it is for my health and well-being. I know that avoiding contact and collision sports is something that I have to do to stay well.

NATHAN KESSEL

My name is Nathan Kessel. I suffered a traumatic brain injury, or concussion, which has changed my life and impacted what I am able to do. I suffered the concussion on July 9, 2009, when I was 12 years old. It happened while attend-ing sailing camp with my two best friends. I was sailing back to the dock and all of a sudden I found myself waking up on the dock and I could see everybody's faces staring at my two bruised, swollen eyes, bloody nose, and bloody fat lip. I panicked because I couldn't focus. There were huge black spots blocking out my vision. My friends told me that someone else had crashed into our boat. The aluminum boom from their boat had swung and hit me across the right side of my head. The impact was so hard that I was launched forward and fell, crush-ing my face on one of the hard fiberglass seats. After I awoke, I was very con-fused; I could not remember anything about sailing or the accident in those first 30 or so minutes after regaining consciousness. The sailing counselor asked me very kindly if I was OK. I said that I wasn't. He called my mom and dad. He was yelling at my mother because she said to call 911 and get me an ambulance and he yelled, "NO, HE'S FINE!"

My friend's mom came to pick me up since my dad was an hour away. My mother was out of town taking care of my ill grandmother, who was hospitalized at the time. I was taken to the emergency department. When I arrived, I was put in a neck brace. The doctors evaluated me. They took X-rays, CAT scans, and an MRI of my head. My mom and brother arrived first, my father, soon after. Miraculously there was nothing broken. I was there for eight hours, waiting and waiting. When I finally returned home late that night, my cousin came over to see how I was feeling. She seemed glad that I was talking. Then she left. Half an hour later my aunt called and told us that my cousin was crying. She was scared and upset because I had no concept of what was going on. I couldn't remember the accident. I didn't remember being at the hospital. I couldn't remember the details of the conversation we were having. I was talking, but not making sense. I went to bed that night with a headache, feeling dizzy.

I slept about twenty hours that night and about twenty hours a day for the next few days, even weeks, which scared my family. After the concussion, I had sensitivity to lights and noise. I had short-term memory loss, frequent severe headaches, dizziness, and confusion. I did strange thing like wash my hands obsessively. I would put items in weird places around the house. When my dad would ask me to put the portable phone on its base, I would put it in anything that had a door. I would put it in the microwave, the cupboard with the dishes, or in the refrigerator. Cell phones, remote controls for the television also would go missing for several days until we were able to find them. I could understand that things should be put away, that they should be put in cabinets. But I couldn't identify a cabinet from an appliance. At first this behavior was quite scary. But now we think that it is hilarious. My brother Sam really helped me by tutoring me and by keeping me laughing, always.

Because of the tremendous support of my incredible pediatrician, Dr. Christine Freemer, I was sent to see Dr. William Meehan at Children's Hospital in Boston, five days after my concussion. Both doctors were adamant that I do as little cognitive activity as possible early on in my recovery. I remained in dim light, whenever possible. I was restricted from participating in swimming, tennis, and strenuous activities. I slept as much as I needed. But it was summer. I wanted to play music, go swimming, play tennis, go bicycling, play video games, go on vacation with my family and hang out with my friends. Dr. Meehan wanted me to recover from the head injury first, and help me get ready to go back to school in two months; to restore my short-term memory, reduce the headaches, and spend more time being wakeful; to help me to become who I once was. So everything was restricted, except hanging out, watching television, listening to music, and talking with my friends!

The first two weeks after my concussion I slept for 20–22 hours at a time; then I would wake up for 30 minutes and go back to sleep. My Bar Mitzvah tutor came to my house two weeks after the concussion to review part of my lesson. She said that I could not do anything because I was taking too long to chant a prayer. I would begin complaining of a headache. So, I had to stop and rest. My mom called Dr. Meehan at the Concussion Clinic. He explained that I could only spend twenty minutes trying to practice my prayers. Then I would develop headaches and sleep for four to six hours. Dr. Meehan always made sure that my mom understood what was happening directly or through his excellent nursing staff.

Dr. Meehan explained that too much cognitive activity was the equivalent of running a marathon. He further explained that I should not be doing cognitive activity because it was like running on a sprained ankle that was constantly being reinjured, never allowing it to fully heal. A concussion affects the brain as though it is sprained. Thinking, reasoning, and other cognitive activities were stressing the brain and causing me to feel exhausted and have headaches, signals from the brain that it was overexerted. Dr. Meehan explained that rehearsing for my Bar Mitzvah was a form of cognitive exertion. He said I needed more time to heal. It was hard to comply as a young, active teenager. But I didn't want to disappoint Dr. Meehan or hinder my progress. So I followed his instructions.

The good thing is I can't remember giving my mom a hard time that first month. I also can't remember that my friends came to visit me during that month. I had a few of my friends over to visit. When we came back inside from playing Frisbee, I have been told I washed my hands for about ten minutes. I am not sure why. I just couldn't stop washing my hands. One of my friends said I was like her grandfather, who has Alzheimer's disease, because I forgot what was going on every five minutes. I had difficulty carrying on a conversation. I needed things repeated constantly. I really don't remember much of that summer.

Things seemed to get back to normal in the fall because of the school routine. But it wasn't easy. When the school year started, I could only go for half days. I would fall asleep in class and then, when it was time to go to my next class, I would go to the wrong one. My friends were so great. They would always help me. I couldn't stay for a full day in the beginning of the year. I needed to do my assignments. But I would sometimes forget to write down my homework. It was my friends who rescued me. The school I attended at the time was not very helpful or cooperative. The principal didn't believe that I needed accommodations as recommended by Dr. Meehan. Some of my teachers were different. They were nice and did try to help. But it was hard for them to believe the symptoms I was suffering and understand my learning difficulties resulted from the concussion. I looked fine. There were no visible indications that I had a concussion. There were no crutches to use, no braces or bandages to wear, no signs that I was healing. There was only documents from Dr. Meehan, his proactive staff, and multiple conversations that fell on deaf ears.

I lived through eighth grade without remembering much of the day-to-day things. My second summer suffering concussive symptoms was the summer before high school. As school had let out for summer, Dr. Meehan recommended another long period of cognitive rest. Well, I had to get creative this time. I had to develop new hobbies and activities. I discovered that I loved golfing. And golf received the stamp of approval from Dr. Meehan. So did bicycling and swimming, without the competitive component. I learned that I have a phenomenal musical proclivity, playing piano, guitar and saxophone well. I was restricted from lessons. But I could listen to anything, and do simple basics playing, as long as it didn't make my symptoms worse.

My concussion has affected me dramatically. I have been forced to repeat and relearn things. But I have learned so many new things that I love to do. Now, I am 14 years old. I recently started high school this fall with a little bump of exhaustion. But Dr. Meehan is available to explain things to me and keep things in perspective. I am still sensitive to loud noises, so I had to drop my favorite course: Concert Band. But my band director is still trying to include me in creative ways. I am also not allowed to be involved in any contact sports, like basketball or volleyball, as I am still recovering.

I know I will have a complete recovery soon. I am truly grateful to my doctors, nurses, and family for their care, patience, and continued support.

SUGGESTED READINGS

Bailes, J., *Sports-Related Concussion.* 1999, St. Louis, MO: Quality Medical Publishing.
Mason, M., *Head Cases: Stories of Brain Injury and Its Aftermath.* 2008, New York: Farrar, Straus and Giroux.
Nowinski, C., *Head Games: Football's Concussion Crisis.* 2007, East Bridgewater, MA: The Drummond Publishing Group.

Appendix: Sports Concussion Assessment Tool (SCAT 2)

SCAT2

 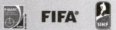

Sport Concussion Assessment Tool 2

Name

Sport/team

Date/time of injury

Date/time of assessment

Age _____   Gender ☐ M   ☐ F

Years of education completed

Examiner

What is the SCAT2?[1]

This tool represents a standardized method of evaluating injured athletes for concussion and can be used in athletes aged from 10 years and older. It supersedes the original SCAT published in 2005[2]. This tool also enables the calculation of the Standardized Assessment of Concussion (SAC)[3,4] score and the Maddocks questions[5] for sideline concussion assessment.

Instructions for using the SCAT2

The SCAT2 is designed for the use of medical and health professionals. Preseason baseline testing with the SCAT2 can be helpful for interpreting post-injury test scores. Words in Italics throughout the SCAT2 are the instructions given to the athlete by the tester.

This tool may be freely copied for distribtion to individuals, teams, groups and organizations.

What is a concussion?

A concussion is a disturbance in brain function caused by a direct or indirect force to the head. It results in a variety of non-specific symptoms (like those listed below) and often does not involve loss of consciousness. Concussion should be suspected in the presence of **any one or more** of the following:

- Symptoms (such as headache), or
- Physical signs (such as unsteadiness), or
- Impaired brain function (e.g. confusion) or
- Abnormal behaviour.

Any athlete with a suspected concussion should be REMOVED FROM PLAY, medically assessed, monitored for deterioration (i.e., should not be left alone) and should not drive a motor vehicle.

Symptom Evaluation

How do you feel?

You should score yourself on the following symptoms, based on how you feel now.

	none	mild		moderate		severe	
Headache	0	1	2	3	4	5	6
"Pressure in head"	0	1	2	3	4	5	6
Neck Pain	0	1	2	3	4	5	6
Nausea or vomiting	0	1	2	3	4	5	6
Dizziness	0	1	2	3	4	5	6
Blurred vision	0	1	2	3	4	5	6
Balance problems	0	1	2	3	4	5	6
Sensitivity to light	0	1	2	3	4	5	6
Sensitivity to noise	0	1	2	3	4	5	6
Feeling slowed down	0	1	2	3	4	5	6
Feeling like "in a fog"	0	1	2	3	4	5	6
"Don't feel right"	0	1	2	3	4	5	6
Difficulty concentrating	0	1	2	3	4	5	6
Difficulty remembering	0	1	2	3	4	5	6
Fatigue or low energy	0	1	2	3	4	5	6
Confusion	0	1	2	3	4	5	6
Drowsiness	0	1	2	3	4	5	6
Trouble falling asleep (if applicable)	0	1	2	3	4	5	6
More emotional	0	1	2	3	4	5	6
Irritability	0	1	2	3	4	5	6
Sadness	0	1	2	3	4	5	6
Nervous or Anxious	0	1	2	3	4	5	6

Total number of symptoms (Maximum possible 22)
Symptom severity score
(Add all scores in table, maximum possible: 22 x 6 = 132)

Do the symptoms get worse with physical activity? ☐ Y ☐ N
Do the symptoms get worse with mental activity? ☐ Y ☐ N

Overall rating
If you know the athlete well prior to the injury, how different is the athlete acting compared to his / her usual self? Please circle one response.

no different	very different	unsure

Cognitive & Physical Evaluation

1 **Symptom score** (from page 1)

22 minus number of symptoms | of 22

2 **Physical signs score**

Was there loss of consciousness or unresponsiveness? ☐ Y ☐ N
If yes, how long? ☐ minutes
Was there a balance problem/unsteadiness? ☐ Y ☐ N

Physical signs score (1 point for each negative response) | of 2

3 **Glasgow coma scale (GCS)**

Best eye response (E)

No eye opening	1
Eye opening in response to pain	2
Eye opening to speech	3
Eyes opening spontaneously	4

Best verbal response (V)

No verbal response	1
Incomprehensible sounds	2
Inappropriate words	3
Confused	4
Oriented	5

Best motor response (M)

No motor response	1
Extension to pain	2
Abnormal flexion to pain	3
Flexion/Withdrawal to pain	4
Localizes to pain	5
Obeys commands	6

Glasgow Coma score (E + V + M) | of 15

GCS should be recorded for all athletes in case of subsequent deterioration.

4 **Sideline Assessment – Maddocks Score**

"I am going to ask you a few questions, please listen carefully and give your best effort."

Modified Maddocks questions (1 point for each correct answer)

At what venue are we at today?	0 1
Which half is it now?	0 1
Who scored last in this match?	0 1
What team did you play last week/game?	0 1
Did your team win the last game?	0 1

Maddocks score | of 5

Maddocks score is validated for sideline diagnosis of concussion only and is not included in SCAT 2 summary score for serial testing.

5 **Cognitive assessment**
Standardized Assessment of Concussion (SAC)

Orientation (1 point for each correct answer)

What month is it?	0 1
What is the date today?	0 1
What is the day of the week?	0 1
What year is it?	0 1
What time is it right now? (within 1 hour)	0 1

Orientation score | of 5

Immediate memory
"I am going to test your memory. I will read you a list of words and when I am done, repeat back as many words as you can remember, in any order."

Trials 2 & 3:
"I am going to repeat the same list again. Repeat back as many words as you can remember in any order, even if you said the word before."

Complete all 3 trials regardless of score on trial 1 & 2. Read the words at a rate of one per second. Score 1 pt. for each correct response. Total score equals sum across all 3 trials. Do not inform the athlete that delayed recall will be tested.

List	Trial 1	Trial 2	Trial 3	Alternative word list		
elbow	0 1	0 1	0 1	candle	baby	finger
apple	0 1	0 1	0 1	paper	monkey	penny
carpet	0 1	0 1	0 1	sugar	perfume	blanket
saddle	0 1	0 1	0 1	sandwich	sunset	lemon
bubble	0 1	0 1	0 1	wagon	iron	insect
Total						

Immediate memory score | of 15

Concentration
Digits Backward:
"I am going to read you a string of numbers and when I am done, you repeat them back to me backwards, in reverse order of how I read them to you. For example, if I say 7-1-9, you would say 9-1-7."

If correct, go to next string length. If incorrect, read trial 2. One point possible for each string length. Stop after incorrect on both trials. The digits should be read at the rate of one per second.

		Alternative digit lists		
4-9-3	0 1	6-2-9	5-2-6	4-1-5
3-8-1-4	0 1	3-2-7-9	1-7-9-5	4-9-6-8
6-2-9-7-1	0 1	1-5-2-8-6	3-8-5-2-7	6-1-8-4-3
7-1-8-4-6-2	0 1	5-3-9-1-4-8	8-3-1-9-6-4	7-2-4-8-5-6

Months in Reverse Order:
"Now tell me the months of the year in reverse order. Start with the last month and go backward. So you'll say December, November ... Go ahead"

1 pt. for entire sequence correct

Dec-Nov-Oct-Sept-Aug-Jul-Jun-May-Apr-Mar-Feb-Jan | 0 1

Concentration score | of 5

[1] This tool has been developed by a group of international experts at the 3rd International Consensus meeting on Concussion in Sport held in Zurich, Switzerland in November 2008. The full details of the conference outcomes and the authors of the tool are published in British Journal of Sports Medicine, 2009, volume 43, supplement 1.
The outcome paper will also be simultaneously co-published in the May 2009 issues of Clinical Journal of Sports Medicine, Physical Medicine & Rehabilitation, Journal of Athletic Training, Journal of Clinical Neuroscience, Journal of Science & Medicine in Sport, Neurosurgery, Scandinavian Journal of Science & Medicine in Sport and the Journal of Clinical Sports Medicine.

[2] McCrory P et al. Summary and agreement statement of the 2nd International Conference on Concussion in Sport, Prague 2004. British Journal of Sports Medicine. 2005; 39: 196-204

[3] McCrea M. Standardized mental status testing of acute concussion. Clinical Journal of Sports Medicine. 2001; 11: 176-181

[4] McCrea M, Randolph C, Kelly J. Standardized Assessment of Concussion: Manual for administration, scoring and interpretation. Waukesha, Wisconsin, USA.

[5] Maddocks, DL; Dicker, GD; Saling, MM. The assessment of orientation following concussion in athletes. Clin J Sport Med. 1995;5(1):32–3

[6] Guskiewicz KM. Assessment of postural stability following sport-related concussion. Current Sports Medicine Reports. 2003; 2: 24-30

6 Balance examination

This balance testing is based on a modified version of the Balance Error Scoring System (BESS)*. A stopwatch or watch with a second hand is required for this testing.

Balance testing

"I am now going to test your balance. Please take your shoes off, roll up your pant legs above ankle (if applicable), and remove any ankle taping (if applicable). This test will consist of three twenty second tests with different stances."

(a) Double leg stance:

"The first stance is standing with your feet together with your hands on your hips and with your eyes closed. You should try to maintain stability in that position for 20 seconds. I will be counting the number of times you move out of this position. I will start timing when you are set and have closed your eyes."

(b) Single leg stance:

"If you were to kick a ball, which foot would you use? [This will be the dominant foot] Now stand on your non-dominant foot. The dominant leg should be held in approximately 30 degrees of hip flexion and 45 degrees of knee flexion. Again, you should try to maintain stability for 20 seconds with your hands on your hips and your eyes closed. If you stumble out of this position, open your eyes and return to the start position and continue balancing. I will start timing when you are set and have closed your eyes."

(c) Tandem stance:

"Now stand heel-to-toe with your non-dominant foot in back. Your weight should be evenly distributed across both feet. Again, you should try to maintain stability for 20 seconds with your hands on your hips and your eyes closed. I will be counting the number of times you move out of this position. If you stumble out of this position, open your eyes and return to the start position and continue balancing. I will start timing when you are set and have closed your eyes."

Balance testing – types of errors
1. Hands lifted off iliac crest
2. Opening eyes
3. Step, stumble, or fall
4. Moving hip into > 30 degrees abduction
5. Lifting forefoot or heel
6. Remaining out of test position > 5 sec

Each of the 20-second trials is scored by counting the errors, or deviations from the proper stance, accumulated by the athlete. The examiner will begin counting errors only after the individual has assumed the proper start position. **The modified BESS is calculated by adding one error point for each error during the three 20-second tests. The maximum total number of errors for any single condition is 10.** If an athlete commits multiple errors simultaneously, only one error is recorded but the athlete should quickly return to the testing position, and counting should resume once subject is set. Subjects that are unable to maintain the testing procedure for a minimum of **five seconds** at the start are assigned the highest possible score, ten, for that testing condition.

Which foot was tested: ▢ Left ▢ Right
(i.e. which is the **non-dominant** foot)

Condition	Total errors
Double Leg Stance (feet together)	of 10
Single leg stance (non-dominant foot)	of 10
Tandem stance (non-dominant foot at back)	of 10
Balance examination score (30 **minus** total errors)	of 30

7 Coordination examination

Upper limb coordination

Finger-to-nose (FTN) task: *"I am going to test your coordination now. Please sit comfortably on the chair with your eyes open and your arm (either right or left) outstretched (shoulder flexed to 90 degrees and elbow and fingers extended). When I give a start signal, I would like you to perform five successive finger to nose repetitions using your index finger to touch the tip of the nose as quickly and as accurately as possible."*

Which arm was tested: ▢ Left ▢ Right

Scoring: 5 correct repetitions in < 4 seconds = 1

Note for testers: Athletes fail the test if they do not touch their nose, do not fully extend their elbow or do not perform five repetitions. Failure should be scored as 0.

Coordination score	of 1

8 Cognitive assessment

Standardized Assessment of Concussion (SAC)

Delayed recall

"Do you remember that list of words I read a few times earlier? Tell me as many words from the list as you can remember in any order."

Circle each word correctly recalled. Total score equals number of words recalled.

List	Alternative word list		
elbow	candle	baby	finger
apple	paper	monkey	penny
carpet	sugar	perfume	blanket
saddle	sandwich	sunset	lemon
bubble	wagon	iron	insect

Delayed recall score	of 5

Overall score

Test domain	Score
Symptom score	of 22
Physical signs score	of 2
Glasgow Coma score (E + V + M)	of 15
Balance examination score	of 30
Coordination score	of 1
Subtotal	**of 70**
Orientation score	of 5
Immediate memory score	of 5
Concentration score	of 15
Delayed recall score	of 5
SAC subtotal	**of 30**
SCAT2 total	**of 100**
Maddocks Score	**of 5**

Definitive normative data for a SCAT2 "cut-off" score is not available at this time and will be developed in prospective studies. Embedded within the SCAT2 is the SAC score that can be utilized separately in concussion management. The scoring system also takes on particular clinical significance during serial assessment where it can be used to document either a decline or an improvement in neurological functioning.

Scoring data from the SCAT2 or SAC should not be used as a stand alone method to diagnose concussion, measure recovery or make decisions about an athlete's readiness to return to competition after concussion.

Athlete Information

Any athlete suspected of having a concussion should be removed from play, and then seek medical evaluation.

Signs to watch for

Problems could arise over the first 24-48 hours. You should not be left alone and must go to a hospital at once if you:

- Have a headache that gets worse
- Are very drowsy or can't be awakened (woken up)
- Can't recognize people or places
- Have repeated vomiting
- Behave unusually or seem confused; are very irritable
- Have seizures (arms and legs jerk uncontrollably)
- Have weak or numb arms or legs
- Are unsteady on your feet; have slurred speech

Remember, it is better to be safe.
Consult your doctor after a suspected concussion.

Return to play

Athletes should not be returned to play the same day of injury. When returning athletes to play, they should follow a stepwise symptom-limited program, with stages of progression. For example:
1. rest until asymptomatic (physical and mental rest)
2. light aerobic exercise (e.g. stationary cycle)
3. sport-specific exercise
4. non-contact training drills (start light resistance training)
5. full contact training after medical clearance
6. return to competition (game play)

There should be approximately 24 hours (or longer) for each stage and the athlete should return to stage 1 if symptoms recur. Resistance training should only be added in the later stages.
Medical clearance should be given before return to play.

Tool	Test domain	Time	Score			
		Date tested				
		Days post injury				
SCAT2	Symptom score					
	Physical signs score					
	Glasgow Coma score (E + V + M)					
	Balance examination score					
	Coordination score					
SAC	Orientation score					
	Immediate memory score					
	Concentration score					
	Delayed recall score					
	SAC Score					
Total	SCAT2					
Symptom severity score (max possible 132)						
Return to play			Y☐ N☐	Y☐ N☐	Y☐ N☐	Y☐ N☐

Additional comments

Concussion injury advice (To be given to concussed athlete)

This patient has received an injury to the head. A careful medical examination has been carried out and no sign of any serious complications has been found. It is expected that recovery will be rapid, but the patient will need monitoring for a further period by a responsible adult. Your treating physician will provide guidance as to this timeframe.

If you notice any change in behaviour, vomiting, dizziness, worsening headache, double vision or excessive drowsiness, please telephone the clinic or the nearest hospital emergency department immediately.

Other important points:
- Rest and avoid strenuous activity for at least 24 hours
- No alcohol
- No sleeping tablets
- Use paracetamol or codeine for headache. Do not use aspirin or anti-inflammatory medication
- Do not drive until medically cleared
- Do not train or play sport until medically cleared

Clinic phone number

Patient's name

Date/time of injury

Date/time of medical review

Treating physician

Contact details or stamp

SCAT2 SPORT CONCUSSION ASSESMENT TOOL 2 | **PAGE 4**

INDEX

About the Author

WILLIAM PAUL MEEHAN, III M.D., is the director of the Sports Concussion Clinic in the Division of Sports Medicine at Children's Hospital Boston. A graduate of Harvard Medical School, Dr. Meehan is board certified in pediatrics, pediatric emergency medicine, and sports medicine. He conducts both clinical and scientific research in the area of concussive brain injury. His research is funded by the National Institutes of Health, the Center for the Integration of Medicine and Innovative Technology, and the National Football League. He has multiple medical and scientific publications. He was the guest editor for the January 2011 edition of *Clinics in Sports Medicine*, which was entirely devoted to the issue of sport-related concussion and serves as ad hoc editor for multiple medical journals.

About the Series Editor

JULIE K. SILVER, M.D., is Assistant Professor, Harvard Medical School, Department of Physical Medicine and Rehabilitation, and is on the medical staff at Brigham & Women's, Massachusetts General, and Spaulding Rehabilitation Hospitals in Boston. Dr. Silver has authored, edited or coedited dozens of books, including medical textbooks and consumer health guides. She is also the chief editor of books at Harvard Health Publications. Dr. Silver has won many awards including the American Medical Writers Association Solimene Award for Excellence in Medical Writing and the prestigious Lane Adams Quality of Life Award from the American Cancer Society. Silver is active teaching health care providers how to write and publish, and she is the director of an annual course offered by the Harvard Medical School Department of Continuing Education titled "Publishing Books, Memoirs and Other Creative Non-Fiction." For more about her work, visit www.JulieSilverMD.com.